MOUNTAIN MIDWIFE

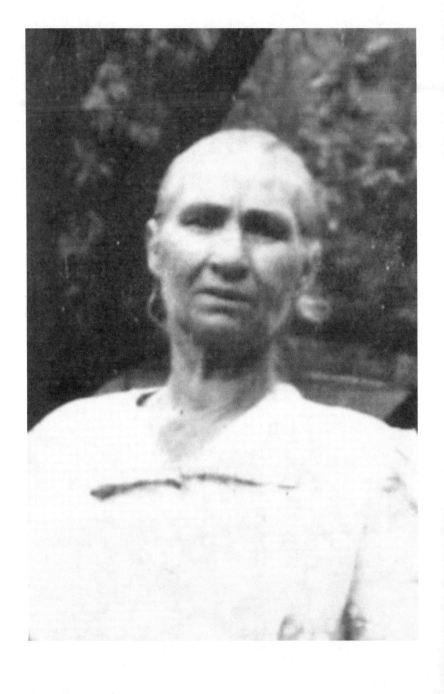

MOUNTAIN MIDWIFE

LIFE AND TIMES OF ISABELLA BROWN NEAL

VICKIE OSBORNE BROWN

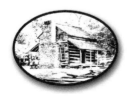

Mountain Memories Books
Charleston, West Virginia

Mountain Memories Books
Charleston, WV

First Edition

10 9 8 7 6 5 4 3 2 1

Printed in the United States of America

Library of Congress Control Number: 2010930798
ISBN-13: 978-0-938985-26-6
ISBN: 0-938985-26-4
Book design: Mark Phillips

Distributed by:

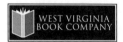

West Virginia Book Company
1125 Central Avenue
Charleston, WV 25302
www.wvbookco.com

TABLE OF CONTENTS

PREFACE

As a young child, Belle had known that she wanted to heal people. Her father, Dr. Anthony Brown, and her uncle, Dr Wash Brown, had doctored the community after their return from the Civil War. Dr. Anthony Brown practiced medicine at an office in Clay. Dr. Wash Brown practiced in the southern part of Clay County, usually riding horseback to see his patients. He had received a bullet wound to his knee during the Civil War and it bothered him until his death. Belle was always around observing and taking part. When she grew older she could see the need for a good midwife and she rose to the challenge. Belle was registered as a Certified Midwife of West Virginia. Her duties were to assist and deliver, keep a log of the birth, and list the parents, their occupations and number of children. She listed the date of the delivery and the sex of a child. She would then take these to the Clay Courthouse where they were recorded at the County Clerk's office. It has been estimated that she delivered 3,000 babies over her career of 40 years or more. Her granddaughter, Chessie, has in her possession some of the books on births that Belle had recorded.

From a very young age Belle had observed and assisted her father with medical situations. She studied child birthing through mail correspondence and received her certificate as a licensed midwife in the 1920s. Through the years she traveled across the mountains and into the valleys to get to her patients. She was a dedicated nurse and midwife, serving those who needed her, especially the poor. She was a pioneer in her lifetime and rejected the custom of the Victorian age when women remained at home.

Belle's world was not large but her talents were many. She stepped up when a medical need arose. She answered to no one and freely spoke her mind. She was called into service no matter the weather or the distance. She was dedicated to her profession, often ignoring her own needs. With the experience gleaned from watching her father doctor the sick, she crisscrossed the mountain trails and paths in daylight or darkness, in hot summers or winter's cold, to get to her patients. Even now when people speak of Belle Neal, they remember her with a smile on her face and a story about her doctoring. She walked and rode her way through the mountains of Clay County with a doctor's bag full of herbs, a lantern and a loaded shotgun. She brought healing and hope to the mountain people of Clay County. In sum, a woman very worthy of recognition.

Isabella Brown was born May 22, 1879 to Dr. Anthony R. Brown and Elizabeth Jarrett Brown. In 1911 she married George Brown Neal and they settled in Charlie's Fork near Bickmore, WV. They moved to land that had previously been owned by her father. They dismantled a house on one side of the road and moved it to where it could be built on a large rock. The previous land would be used as a garden. The year they moved in the house, George and Belle welcomed their first child, Glacie, in November. In the following years Belle gave birth to more children: Gladie, Radar, John O, Ralph, Ray and one adopted son, Lester Leo Jarrett.

Belle was the youngest child of the Browns. Her sisters were Martha, who married James Henry Osborne, and Cordelia, who married John R. Neal. Her brothers were John and Irvin. Belle's descendants are scattered across Clay County to this day.

BELLE'S 60th BIRTHDAY

It was near midnight, the peepers were calling, and the house had finally cooled down enough so a body could sleep. It was quiet in this little isolated holler where Belle lived. She could hear the trees swaying as a slight breeze ruffled the new leaves. Belle was just drifting off as she heard the fall of running feet hit her porch and the call of "Aunt Belle, Aunt Belle." Knowing there would be no sleep tonight she felt her way to the door, not bothering to light the lantern, for there was urgency in the voice at the door.

When she pulled back the bar on the door and let it swing wide she could see the startled face of young ten-year old Homer. He held his lantern high and his blue eyes were huge in his face; his rumpled blonde hair stood on end. His overalls, too short in the legs, were hooked by one strap, and his feet were bare. Between gasps of breath he said, "Aunt Belle, Mony said to come quick as you can. She needs you." Realizing that he was close to hysterics, she pulled him into the room and spoke in a calming voice.

"Alright Homer, you come in and have some cornbread and a glass of buttermilk while I gather my things. Rildy will be all right till I get there. She knows what to do—this bein' her ninth child. You need to catch your breath before we start back down the mountain and I need to change out of my night clothes."

The calming voice must have reassured him because Homer set his lantern down and went over to the table as Aunt Belle poured him a fresh cup of buttermilk from the crock on the table. He could hear Uncle George snoring in his sleep over in his corner bed. Uncle George was so accustomed to people waking Belle in the middle of the night that it did not disturb his sleep. Homer helped himself to a large piece of cornbread while Belle gathered her medical bag and changed her clothes. When he had nearly finished his milk,

Belle said, "Come now Homer, and hold the light while I saddle Old Boss."

They waded through the damp grass to a shed where Belle kept her horse. Homer held the light high and Belle took the blanket and saddle from the rail. As she worked, she questioned Homer about Marilda's condition, "Are her pains close? Who's with her now?"

"Well, Pap was there and Forest went to get Grandma Annie. And Annie Exline was there too. Pap said for me to come through the woods since it was faster and tell you to come on; he's no good with child birthing," Homer said.

Belle continued to talk as she settled the saddle and buckled it beneath the horse, after checking to make sure the cinch was tight. She tied her well-worn doctor's bag over the saddle horn. "She'll be alright son. Don't worry; Annie knows what to do if her time comes 'fore I get there. Take my hand now and get up behind me," she instructed as she hoisted herself up from a tree stump she kept in the shed.

Homer grabbed her hand and jumped up behind her on the horse. He held on tight as Belle set off at a fast pace back up the mountain road that she could travel in the dark or with her eyes closed.

Old Boss was used to these midnight travels and plopped along at a fast pace as Belle nudged the horse up the steep mountain road. Boss was an old horse, but her determination was evident in the way she held her head, her ears perked for any sounds that might present danger. For her dedication, Belle gave her an affectionate pat when they reached the crossroads at the top of the mountain where four roads met. Off in the distance of Beechy Ridge, Belle and Homer heard the shrill cry of a mountain lion and Old Boss shivered. "Easy Boss," Belle coaxed as she patted her neck, "ain't no cat goin' get us tonight. We got a new youngin' comin' into the world."

A sliver of moon sent down an eerie light as it rocked in the clear sky. Homer could hear the baritone barks of coon dogs vibrating and echoing as they bounced off the high mountain walls. "I believe Marv Brown's dogs have got something treed," said Homer.

"Sounds like," replied Belle, "he's got near 14 head of dogs; they must all be out tonight."

Belle kicked Boss into a faster pace as they started down a steep hill. Homer clung with security to Aunt Belle's waist as they headed down the mountain toward home. She smelled like tobacco and the fresh scent of sun-dried clothes, both a comforting smell to Homer. A little ways down the mountain road they turned to the right and down a steep narrow trail. Belle could see the lights shining dimly through the windows of the upper room of the clapboard house as shadows played across the drawn curtains. Spring peepers broke the stillness of the mountains and the scent of new blooms penetrated their nostrils as the breeze blew a cooling wave here near the creek.

On down the holler Belle could see a light at Okey's house shining from the back bedroom. Belle thought one of the youngin's must be sick and Deretha was probably up tendin' to them. Belle thought to herself she would probably be agoin' there soon, for Deretha was expectin' again.

"Whoa there, whoa there, Boss," she called to the old horse as they approached the house. She gave Homer a hand down from behind her and, handing him her doctor bag, she slid down to the ground.

Forest, a young man of thirteen, sat on the porch looking anxious. He held another light high as Belle came across the yard. Little Ruth was in the kitchen stirrin' up the fire and Bib was bringing water from the spring. Homer led Old Boss to the barn to remove her saddle and put her up for the night. With a clean gunnysack, he wiped the old horse down and gave her a little water.

Belle stepped through the door of the house and saw that Clem and John were both sleeping over in the corner bed in the livin' room. She could hear Bib's mother, Annie Osborne, talking from the back bedroom and she headed that way. As Belle set down the medical bag, Annie Osborne turned from where she had been wiping Marilda's face, "It's about time you got here, Belle! I thought me and Annie Exline might have to deliver this one ourselves."

As Belle cleaned her hands from a basin of water on the dresser, she turned to Annie Osborne and Annie Exline. "Now you know I always make it in time to catch the babies; besides, Homer come runnin' fast as he could for a boy in the night. Rildy knows what to do anyway; long as there is no trouble, she could have done it on her own. Annie how ye been, have you been delivering many babies?" Belle asked as she scrubbed her hands and got ready to examine Marilda.

Annie Exline said, "I have delivered a few by myself, but I like to look in when someone is doing a delivery. I want to get as much experience as possible for when I have to go it alone."

"Well I'm glad you're here anyways. I got Ruth out of bed to help me and Bib is carryin' water. I decided to let Clem and Johnny sleep," said Grandma Annie.

Just then Marilda gave a deep moan as she writhed in pain and Belle rushed to her side. Soothing her head with her hand after checking to see how far she had dilated, Belle said, "It won't be to much longer now, child. Just a couple good pushes and it'll all be over. Ya'll keep the kids outside, and Bib too! I can handle the rest and Annie Exline is here if I need her."

Grandma Annie silently left the room with a shake of her head, glad that Belle was here to handle the birth. She could have done it, but Belle was better. She could do more good by praying anyway, so she went to the bed where the boys still slept and knelt down to ask God's mercy for Marilda and the new babe.

Belle talked in a soothing voice as she calmed the expectant mother. Then she pressed and massaged the stomach, helping to coax the child from the birth canal. When the baby was delivered, she laid the child on Marilda's stomach and cut the cord with a pair of sterilized scissors that she kept in her doctor's bag. Annie stayed right by Belle's side. She was a good student.

Sometime later Grandma heard the first cries of her newest grandchild ringing loudly through the quiet house. She thought it would wake the boys, but they slept on. Grandma went to the bedroom door and Belle smiled as she handed her the new baby, then went back to work on Marilda. Belle forced the afterbirth and placed it in a cloth for burning. After placing clean linens beneath Marilda and wrapping her in a clean quilt, she began to gather her medical supplies.

Grandma wrapped the crying baby girl in a warm blanket and soothed back the head of black hair from her face. "Rildy will be glad for another girl among all these boys," she thought as she carried her to the kitchen to bathe her with some warm water and rub warm oil over her body.

After she cleaned the little girl up, she placed a band around the stomach and pinned it to keep the cord in place. Seven-year-old Ruth already had the warm water poured and a clean rag on the kitchen table.

Ruth said, "Grandma, is it another snotty-nosed boy?"

Grandma shook her head and smiled as she said, "No, Ruthie, you've got a sister now to help you fight all them boys."

"I hope she helps me clean and cook; these boys sure make a mess for one girl to work on."

Grandma said, "Them boys had better not dirty up this kitchen you have worked so hard on."

Ruth liked it when Grandma took her side on things. They both wondered what the baby's name would be but no one had spoken of that yet. Ruth said she didn't care what name they gave her as long as she had a girl to play with. They both admired the now squalling baby as Grandma placed her in a new gown. After wrapping her in a flannel blanket, they headed for the porch where Bib and the boys waited.

Grandma Annie handed Bib the new baby in one hand while he held his Prince Albert cigarette in the other. Homer and Forest crowded around to see the baby, who had settled down and was sucking her thumb. "That sure is one ugly baby," said Homer.

"Is it a boy or girl?" asked Forest.

"It's a new baby sister," Grandma said.

"What's her name Pap?" asked Ruth.

"I think we'll call her Annie after Ma and Annie Exline who helped with the birth."

"You mean take Grandma Osborne's name?" said Ruth.

Forest and Homer giggled and Forest said, "No silly! Just call her the same as Grandma."

Grandma laughed and said, "That's a good name for her, but I bet she'll curse that head of wiry hair. We'll have to keep it pinned up to keep it out of her face." They all laughed at that.

Just then Belle came out on the porch and wiped her face with a damp cloth. "Well, Rildy is sleeping now. Ms. Osborne, you can take over from here. I need to get home; I have to sterilize my medical instruments and I could use some sleep. What did you name the baby, Bib?"

Homer said, "We're goin' call her Anne after Grandma Annie."

"Well that's a good name, but I would have liked to have her named after me. I got to get home, but I'll be back in the morning to check on Rildy," said Belle as she scurried down the steps and with a wave she went to get her horse.

Forest laughed and said, "Anne Belle, now that's some name!"

Homer went to saddle Old Boss for Belle and she thanked him and waved goodbye as she headed toward home. The night was balmy and the soothing night sounds seemed to enclose the hills along the little holler as Belle rode toward home. Night birds called from the darkness. Nearly a full moon cast ghostly shadows down on the little settlement. Clouds looking like large puffs of cotton rolled across the sky and played hiding with the moon.

Belle wondered how many babies this one made that she had helped bring into the world. "Well all is safe now," she told herself as she gazed up at the sky seeing the brightness of the stars and feeling alone in the world, just herself and the Big Dipper. "It seems that I am alone in the world on these long rides in the night," thought Belle. It was May 22, 1937, and Belle had just spent her 60th birthday doing what she did best—another baby brought safely into the world. So goes the life of a mountain midwife.

As she nudged Old Boss to her shed, she thought she and Old Boss were both getting too old for nightly tramps. She struggled to touch the ground with her feet and retrieve her doctor's bag. Dawn would soon break across the sky so Belle hurried to remove the saddle from the old horse. She gave her an extra scoop of oats and a couple of pats as she turned toward the house.

"Mornings come too early," thought Belle as she rustled her old body out of the bed and stretched to remove the kinks from her neck after only a few hours' sleep. She headed toward the spring with her water bucket. She liked her coffee made with fresh-drawn water. She looked out over her little farm as she walked toward the spring, thinking how she liked living here at the foot of the mountains where two small branches met and ran right by her front steps. Nothing could lure a body to sleep like clear, cold gurgling water from a small stream.

As she walked along she thought that they needed to get their taters in the ground soon; the leaves were already bigger than a squirrel's ear. Maybe she'd get Radar to lay off the tater rows today. She could see lettuce and onions peeking through the ground. She just couldn't wait for a good mess of wilted lettuce. Even the wild greens of poke, wild lettuce and beets she had been cooking didn't satisfy her like fresh home-grown lettuce.

She was going to ask Forest and Homer to gather some Virginia snakeroot for her while they were out in the woods. She brewed up a tea from the herb and bottled it to make a good tonic. She depended on snakeroot more than any other plant.

So many spring herbs, "bitters," were now ready to be harvested and Belle didn't know if she would have time to gather all she needed. Sometimes the kids would gather herbs they knew she used and leave them on her porch. "There was sure some good kids around here," she thought.

She stayed busy delivering babies and now people along Middle Creek had begun to call on her for other medical needs. People couldn't travel the ten miles to Clay to get a doctor anytime one was needed; most didn't have money for a doctor, anyway.

Belle's father, Anthony, and her Uncle Wash had served in the Civil War. Anthony joined when he was 14 years old and served with the 7th WV regiment. Wash, who joined the 7th WV regiment at 18 years of age, rose to the rank of captain near the end of the war. They came back to Clay County to take up the medical needs of the community. They had been called on for all types of injury and illness—from epidemics, mining accidents or childbirth. If needed, they applied their self-training, even if pressed into service beyond their experience.

Since there was usually no time, means, or money to reach a doctor or hospital, Anthony and Wash were most of the backwood's people only hope. Some they saved, but the mortality rate was high in the backwoods during this time. Doctors and midwives were revered and respected by all, since sickness and tragedy came to all.

The morning sun had finally reached down to warm the little holler where Belle lived. As she returned to the house with her fresh-drawn water, steam rose from the dew-kissed grass and the water gurgled from the small stream as it passed across the rocky bottom. Her old jersey cow mooed to be milked, "Hush up old girl. I'll get to you soon enough."

Songbirds stirred as they awakened to a new day and their muted songs penetrated the silence. Winters were cold here in this little holler and sometimes Belle wished for a home on the mountain. But when spring arrived, gracing the hills, hollers, and trees with pink, yellow, purple and green, there was no place she would rather be.

Belle poured the water into her blue granite coffee pot and measured out the fresh grounds of Eight O'clock coffee from her 5 lb can. She worked quickly; setting the pot over the fire she had started in the cook stove. She grabbed her favorite white enameled mixing bowl from the cupboard, got three cups of flour from the cabinet that had been her mother's, and began to mix the flour. Throwing in a pinch of salt, soda and buttermilk, mixing mostly with her hands and turning it out on the floured table, she soon slid a large pan of biscuits into the hot oven.

She heard stirring from the backroom and looked up just as Radar came thru the door hooking up his overalls. "Ma, why didn't you wake me earlier? You know I like to cook the breakfast."

Not taking time to stop, she began to slice bacon as she talked, "Well Radar, I need to get down to Rildy's this morning and check on her and the new baby. I got lots to do today."

"You mean Rildy has another baby. Seems like they had enough already," he said as he began to crack eggs in a bowl and stir them.

"Yell, well that ain't up to me now is it? Only Rildy and God."

"Humph," said Radar as he placed a big iron skillet on the stove.

"Me and George need to get some things from the store when I get done at Rildy's. I need to check the post office, too. I ordered me a new knife to cut the 'bibilical cord and I hope it is there. You stay here and lay off the rows for our tator bed. I got to get them in the ground; leaves are as big as squirrel's ears now. I'm going out and get some of my silver I keep hid in the Mason jar. It sure is getting low. Most people just pay me with meal and such for doctoring, but I need to make some hard earned cash. I hope George gets that job down at the mines soon."

Radar didn't answer; knowing he wasn't expected to, he just kept tending to breakfast. George soon roused when he smelled the coffee and bacon. He stretched and groaned as he brought his old body, stooped and bent, from the bed. His gray hair, bristly and thick, stood on end. He placed his feet on the cool floor. "Where's your Ma?" he asked Radar as he yawned and stretched again.

"She's out at the cellar counting her money, said she was a goin' to the store," Radar said as he pulled the golden brown biscuits from the oven.

"Guess she'll be a wantin' me to walk to the store with her," George spoke more to himself than to Radar. He grumbled and moaned as he hitched up his suspenders and shifted across the wood floor with his head down and pulled out a kitchen chair. Radar poured George a cup of hot steaming coffee and placed a pitcher of cream nearby, then turned to the stove to take up the crisp bacon.

George sipped his coffee and smacked his lips, still yawning and stretching as he did every morning while he waited for Radar to dish up his breakfast.

"I hate to walk all the way to the store today, my rheumatism is actin' up again," George said, as he buttered his hot biscuits.

As George and Radar finished breakfast, Belle came in and poured herself a hot cup of black coffee. Radar stopped and dished up her breakfast.

"What did Rildy have this time?" asked George.

"Thisn' is a girl," said Belle, "I was a hopin' she'd name it for me, but she called her Annie after Bib's ma."

"How many youngin's that make Bib and Marilda?" asked George.

"Well, she's birthed nine now, but only five was a livin'. Her first one was stillborn—a little girl, then Zela lived about six months. After that Forest was born, then Little Vance—he sure was a smart little tad, talked like a politician. Then Homer was born in '27. That winter Vance came down with what we all thought was the whooping cough. It was in December and Bib was agoin' huntin'. While he was in the woods, Vance took a turn for the worse. Bib, known' something was wrong, came in from the woods and they got someone to take them to the hospital heading for Charleston. That youngin' didn't make it but to Clendenin. It went awful hard on Bib; he couldn't go to the table and eat for months without thinking of Vance. Rildy said he'd come to the table and look at Vance's place with tears a rollin' down his cheeks, then get up and leave the house. That nearly broke Bib," said Belle.

"Well, I know they had lost a few babies, but it happens all the time," George said as he finished up his breakfast. "What time you plannin' on leavin' today, Belle?"

"I'm goin' help Radar start on the tator patch and then wash up some and change my clothes. About two hours from now I can be ready to go."

"I'll be ready," said George, "While we're down that way I'm aimin' to see if that job has come through at the mines."

Two hours later found Belle and George walking down the mountain road that had been dug out by hand by George's brother John. They admired the blooms on the cherry trees in the orchard along the road; it looked for certain like John would have a good crop of cherries this year. George was thinking how John was always working at something. John worked several gardens in the holler, had orchards on all the hilltops, kept gasoline to sell, and worked the road from Route 16 to his house with a mule and a log attached to level the ground. He pedaled vegetables and fruit along Middle Creek. He built his barn and outbuildings with precision and care. When called on to build a chimney from cut stones, he was always ready. John kept his tools in top-notch shape, sharpened and oiled. He liked his land mowed, his trees trimmed and his house in good repair. George never could figure where John got all that ambition!

When Belle and George got to the house, Belle found Marilda sitting up in bed nursing the baby. Belle took the baby and burped her, then lifted her and said she must weigh about seven pounds. After checking to see that Dilly had the cord banded correctly, she handed the new baby over to her sister Dilly and began to check on her patient.

Belle massaged Marilda's stomach to be certain no afterbirth remained and then she packed her with sterile linen pads that had been baked in the oven. She warned Marilda that she must remain in bed a few days and rest before she took her leave. Belle just couldn't resist teasing Marilda though, "Rildy, I thought for certain you would name this baby after me since she arrived on my 60th birthday," Belle said with a grin.

"Well, you know I would have, Aunt Belle, but Bib had his heart set on givin' her his mommy's name."

"And so it will be," said Belle as she left the porch and went to get her old horse.

THE COUNTRY STORE

Belle and George walked the mile to the Bickmore post office with Belle in the lead and George following behind with his back bent and his face toward the ground. People who saw them pass by would shake their heads and smile. Belle checked at the post office and was happy to see that the bone-handled knife she had ordered had finally arrived.

George said he would go to the mines and check on his job. Belle remained at the post office and visited with neighbors and relatives who came by. Just about everyone knew Belle. Some asked advice on an illness or would tell her that they would need her soon for a new delivery. "Well you know where we live, don't ye?" was all Belle would say. George came back from the mine office and told Belle that he would start the new job on Monday; Belle was relieved.

Belle and George started walking along the road to the grocery store when their nephew, Hal, came along in his new truck and told them he would give them a ride to the store. Belle got in the front with Hal and George hoisted himself into the bed.

Hal said, "How you doing, Aunt Belle?"

"Well, we're fit as a fiddle," Belle said, "Now Hal don't be drivin' fast; I'm nervous of anything that goes faster than a horse."

Hal just laughed, but he knew that Belle meant what she said.

"I'm planning on going to the bank in Clay soon, Aunt Belle. Do you need to go?"

"Yell I do. When are ye fixin' to go? That's a right smart way for me and George to walk."

"Well," said Hal, "how about tomorrow morning? I'll drop you off at the drug store while I go to the bank." "Sure," said Belle, "Me and George can be down at the Bickmore Bridge by 8 o'clock in the morning."

"Well that will be just fine. I'll be along about then," said Hal. As they were getting out of the truck, Belle stopped to thank Hal for the ride. "Say, Hal, do you think you could take me and George home today? I might buy a little extra if I don't have to carry it home on my back."

"Why, sure, Aunt Belle. Go on in and order your groceries. I'll drive you as far as I can, and then we'll get your horse and sled and carry everything on home. Don't forget your chewing tobacco and Mickey Twist; I know you and George both like your tobacco."

"Yell, we might be able to afford a little since George got his job at the mines and I'm awful glad of it too," said Belle.

George and Belle stepped inside the grocery store and waited for their eyes to adjust to the darkness. It was a lot cooler inside too. The clerk was sitting in a rocker at the old potbellied stove and Belle's nephew, Owen, was behind the counter writing up a bill.

"Well, hello Aunt Belle and Uncle George," said the clerk, "I been expectin' you all for a week or more. How have you been? Got any news?"

"Yell, Rildy had her baby last night; it was a girl and everything is fine."

"I'm glad. There are so many people moving in along Middle Creek; I expect you'll be busy delivering babies all the time. Most are comin' in to work the mines; blacks, Chinese, Italians, lots of poor folks moving into the company houses. You know they won't be able to afford a doctor."

"Well, I guess me, Annie Exline and Maggie Legg will be kept busy. I was called on to go into Kanawha County and Nicholas too. I'm gettin' too old now to keep up that schedule; sometimes they come and get me in a vehicle, but most of the time I have to ride Old Boss. I hate to tell people no when I see they are in need of a granny midwife."

"I'm goin' to need to place my grocery order," Belle said. "Hal is goin' take me and George home."

"You tell me what you need, Aunt Belle", said the store clerk, "And I'll pack it up for you."

"Okay," said Belle, "I need 50 lbs flour, 25 lbs corn meal, 10 lbs pinto beans, 2 bars castile soap, a cloverine salve, 1 lb raisins, 1lb prunes, 5 lbs Hills Brothers coffee or the Eight O'clock one, horseradish seeds, a bottle of Black Draught, some safety pins, 3 yards of red checkered gingham and a bottle of Watkins vanilla. Was you wanting anything in particular, George?"

"Don't forget our tobacco," said George as he sat rocking by the stove.

"Yell we'd better take 2 pouches of Mail Pouch and 1 Mickey Twist," said Belle as she went to the pop cooler and took out a root beer for George and a Nehi grape for herself. "Put these on our order too, girl," said Belle. Then she went over to sit by George, drinking their cold drinks and visiting with everyone who came in the store.

A TRIP TO CLAY

Belle was waiting at the Bickmore Bridge early the next day, when Hal pulled up and she hoisted her petite form into the front of the truck.

"Where's Uncle George today?" asked Hal.

"Oh that trip yesterday 'bout done him in, he's a-restin' up to start that job at the mines Monday. Besides, he knows I'm goin' because I need some medical supplies and he don't want to sit and wait."

"Uncle George is a goin' to work at the Ward Mines? You know that I work in the office there, so I'll be writin' his paycheck," Hal said with humor.

"Yell, I'll be the one comin to pick up his paycheck. What day do you do the payroll? Don't short him any or I'll be comin' in to complain," Belle said emphatically.

Hal had to laugh at Belle's attitude and said, "Now you know I wouldn't do that, but don't stir up any hard feelings, Aunt Belle."

Hal kept his new truck at a snail's pace as they traveled down Route 16. There were so many potholes and so many people walking along the road. Few had cars and most walked to work or school. Every company house along the road seemed to overflow with children.

Different nationalities living in such close proximity often caused trouble. The company houses were built in rows, one identical to the other. There were no luxuries, no inside plumbing, only one stove for heating the whole house, all weathered and rough wood that no one took the time to paint. At every spot flat enough to build a shack, there was a small house built. The old gob piles were smoking and burning all over the mountains, giving off an acid smell that hung over the camp.

Everyone had to walk to a community well and carry their

drinking water. Many women took their kettles and washboards down along the creek to do their laundry. Almost every house had lines stretched across the front porch to hang their wash. Coal piles marred the yards of every home and clutter was present at every turn. Life was hard on everyone these years following the Depression, but it must have been hardest on those who knew very little English. Coal camps were similar wherever they moved. Mountain people were most hesitant about changes or lifestyles. They were leery to welcome strangers to their way of living.

About all that the new people could call their own were a few pieces of beat up furniture and a parcel of youngins. The foreigners were so new to this way of life and desperate for work to provide for their families that they did whatever it took to get work.

Vegetation grew sparsely on the mountains. Children kept the grass beaten on the yards and the sulfur odor of burning coal floated through the air. It seemed that everything was covered with a film of coal dust. Blasts from the mines shook the foundations of the homes, and the roads were always busy with the comings and goings of the workers and their families.

The train spur that connected with the B&O Railroad at the Elk River ran several trips through the community on what people called the Jitney. Little children at play would stop and wave at the vehicles as they passed. Belle shook her head as she watched, knowing that most of these children would struggle their entire lives.

Coal camp houses were usually built poorly, with wide cracks in the floor and walls. How well they ate depended on how much work their daddy got at the mines. Many would never make it past childhood, due to poverty, illness, and poor sanitation. But for those who did survive, they would no doubt live a life just as hard as the generation before them.

The boys became men quickly, as most were sent into the mines when they were in their teens to help make a living for a large family. When the work played out at one mine, many families moved on to new camps looking for work and a means of survival. Most never stayed anywhere long enough to call a place home or to get to know the locals. Belle had tended to many of these people and she knew of their struggles.

Hal drove slowly through the graveled streets of Clay. The streets were full of people and much activity was going on everywhere in town. Hal stopped across the street from the emporium. Belle hitched up her skirts as she climbed out of the truck, "Where do you want me to meet you at Hal, and how long will you be?"

"I have some business at the bank and the courthouse. Do you want to meet me down at the Big Star Cafe about noon?" Hal asked.

"That will be fine with me. I'll just go on in and visit awhile and get my supplies till then," said Belle as she closed the door. "I might be seein' a lot of people I ain't seen in awhile and they will be wantin' to chew the fat."

Hal just shook his head and laughed at Aunt Belle. She was wearing a dress with an apron made from feed sacks, clean but wrinkled, and a pair of high top canvas shoes. Her red socks peeped above her canvas shoes. He pulled away and Belle crossed the street and entered the drugstore. Only two people were waiting, so Belle took a seat. "How's things on Middle Creek these days, Belle? Are ye busy deliverin' babies?" asked the druggist.

"I sure am. Can't even get my garden planted and I delivered a new baby for Rildy this week."

"Well, I knew she was expectin'. I saw Bib in town two weeks ago. Is she doing all right? I used to love havin' her work here for me; don't get to see her much now."

"She's doin' fine, but with six youngin's to raise along with a garden, she'll be out there working soon enough."

"I'll be needin' some medicine from ye and some advice on how to lance a boil," said Belle. "Old Widder Holcomb asked me at the post office the other day which was best to open a boil. Said she had one on her buttock and was too embarrassed to ask a man what to do, so I thought I'd let her know. I told her to sit in some warm water and it might help to draw the pus out."

Mr. Stephenson said, "Yell that will work. Then tell her after she gets it open to keep it drained and mix sulfur and petroleum jelly

into a paste and keep it covered."

"There is a woman on Beechy Ridge that is expectin' a baby and she's got a goiter on her neck. I want to get some potassium iodine for her. That is the best they is for goiters!"

"Yell, here's a little that will do ye for awhile, Belle. I have got to order some drugs this week and I'll put that on my order."

"Did you know your brother John is runnin' for office again?"

"No," barked Belle, "and I don't want to know anything about him. He doesn't seem to know me unless he wants a vote for something!"

"Now Belle, you just take things the wrong way; you and John never did hit it off," laughed Doc Stephenson.

"The last time he run for office, he run into me and George in town—come along with a big grin on his face—and I said, "Don't ask me to vote for ye!" I pointed to a dog goin' down the street. 'I'd rather kiss that dog's ass with the piles than vote for you," I told him and he left in a huff. I meant it too!

"I'm agoin' walk down the street to the Big Star," she told the doc, "and Hal said he'd buy my lunch. Thanks for the medicine and I'll see ye when I get into town again. It's been a long time since breakfast this mornin' and I am a gettin' hungry."

She stopped along the way as she met people on the street to catch up on the latest news. So many people were in town—this being Saturday—and they seemed to come in droves. Many were walking on the street; some with babies in their arms and a small herd of kids following along behind.

Men gathered in groups, talking loudly and spitting tobacco juice in the street. Men and women, looking too old for their years, walked along the streets carrying the smaller youngins' and a whole brood behind them. It was not unusual to see a woman's bare breast along the street as she fed a baby. They came to town to get things they could not purchase at the company store.

Finally Belle arrived at the Big Star Cafe in the middle of town. It was a busy place this time of day but she finally found a table where she could sit. Belle ordered the special of the day and sipped hot coffee while she waited for the food. "How's George doing, Belle? I ain't seen him in town for a while," some man asked.

"Well he's fair to middlin', I guess. You know George—he grumbles a lot. I don't pay him much mind. And I guess he'll be going to work on Monday at the mines and none too soon, either! Cash is gettin' low around our place but people are good to trade me some food items when I doctor, even though most don't have enough for their selves.

Belle continued, "I guess you heard about Hal a havin' a family reunion out at his place? He's inviting everyone around—about all's kin to us anyways. I hope that ole Sis doesn't show up! I'll give her a piece of my mind! She was always so mean to my mother," Belle said with a snarl on her face, "You think you might make it over? There will be plenty of family comin' too."

"I don't know Belle. Times it's hard for me to travel that far, but I might if I don't have to work that day. I have to work everyday I can."

One woman asked Belle if she would come and stay for the layin' in of her baby. Belle assured her that she would but they would have to send someone to fetch her. Belle said, "I ain't as spry as I used to be. I have to ride a horse or go by car."

Hal came in and ordered the Blue Plate Special and sat drinking strong black coffee as he waited for his food. They had finished their meal and were about to leave when a young shy girl approached Belle. "Ms. Neal, I heard you are real good at curin' sick babies."

"Well I have cured quite a few. You got a sick baby, girl?"

"Yes Ma'am. He is only two weeks old. The granny woman that delivered him said he was too weak and wouldn't live long. He cries a lot and cain't suck the tit. I don't know what else to do. Would you take him and try to help him?"

"Now girl, you go home and git that youngin' and I'll take him home and care for him a few days. Maybe I can pull him through this."

The young girl was so relieved; she wrung her hands and smiled as she told Belle, "Oh, I just know you can save him! I'll go get him ready and bring him back."

"Only the good Lord knows that, girl, but I'll use the knowledge He gave me. Go on now and get him ready," she said as she patted the girl's arm, "I'm a fixin' to go home soon."

While the girl was gone, Hal said he would wait for Belle in the truck just outside the café. The girl was back in quick time. She had a little baby boy bundled and a sack of clothes to send along.

"He sure is a puny little thing ain't he?" Belle examined the baby and said she believed he had a cleft palate. "He needs milk in small portions, like feedin' a baby bird. You come get him in two weeks. We'll know by then. What's his name?"

"I call him Benjamin for his granddaddy," said the girl as she kissed the baby goodbye and handed him to Belle. The young mother left with a broken heart, but she knew if anyone could pull him through, it would be Belle.

Hal saw Belle walking along, carrying a baby and a sack over her shoulder; he helped get her in the truck. "Looks like you got a sick child there, Aunt Belle," said Hal.

"Yell, I'm goin' to try and save this little feller's life," she said as they drove slowly through town. "I'll need to stop at the druggist and get a nasal dropper to feed this youngin' with."

"Well I'll go over to the farm store and pick up some things I need there while you are gone," Hal told her. He just shook his head, thinking, "You never know what Belle will bring home next!"

Hal drove at a crawl up the mountain avoiding rocks to get to Belle's home. When they got to the top of the mountain, he stopped and told Belle she would have to walk down the other side that was rocky and rutted from recent rains. He helped Belle out of the car, picked up her belongings, and carried them to her home while she stepped carefully with the baby.

Belle placed the baby on the table and began to examine his little body. He fretted constantly because he was so hungry. Belle heated warm milk and added a few drops of an herb she used to soothe a small stomach. She fed the baby very slowly by placing the dropper into the side of his mouth. Once the baby got the hang of it he was able to take in 4 ounces of milk. Belle burped and rocked the baby until he slept. She laid him on the bed in the corner and began to put away her purchases.

Radar came in from outside, hot and sweaty.

"Did you get them tators in the ground, Radar?" Belle asked, as she kept busy putting the house in order.

"Yell Ma, Forest came up to visit and he helped me cover them."

"Yell Forest is a mighty fine boy. Him and Homer both are good workers. They will help Bib work and raise the rest of the family. That's the way our family has always been—we help one another when the needs arise," said Belle. "If you can't depend on your relatives to help ye, you don't have much of a family is what I always think."

CARING FOR LITTLE BEN

It was 5 a.m. and Belle had been up every two hours feeding a baby with an eyedropper. His cries were so pitifully weak that he sounded like a baby kitten and seemed to be slowly starving to death. Belle would hold him close and rock him until he would fall asleep. Belle finally dropped off to sleep patting the baby.

When Radar got up to fix breakfast, he found Belle sitting in the rocker with her head drooped to one side, but the baby was safe and fast asleep in her arms.

Radar began to prepare the breakfast as quietly as he could, knowing that Belle needed to sleep.

He filled the big blue granite coffee pot with coffee and water and set it on the back of the stove. He decided to fix a stack of flapjacks. While they were sizzling in the big iron skillet, he went to the cellar for some maple syrup they had made during the winter. When the aroma of fresh coffee and flapjacks penetrated the house, Belle and George both began to stir. Belle gently laid the little baby on her bed and patted him until he rested. After covering him with a warm blanket she stumbled to the kitchen table.

During the next two weeks Belle cared for the baby and taught him to eat from the dropper. She bathed, pampered, and cared for his every need. Due to her care, little Ben began to thrive. Belle rocked him to sleep each night, and carried him on her hip through the day.

Two weeks after handing Ben over to Belle, Rose arrived to take her baby home. She was so glad to see how the baby had grown, when she didn't even know if he would still be alive! She cradled and patted the baby while Belle told her how to care for him. When she had gathered the baby's belongings, she hugged Belle, and with tears in her eyes she said, "I will never forget this good deed you done for me, Ms. Neal. I will be beholden to you forever." She waved goodbye and went to catch her ride home, as Belle stood on the porch waving with tears in her eyes. She would miss the little Ben.

A WET SPRING

Blackberry summer arrived and everything was cold and wet. The old saying was that if it rained on the blackberry bloom on the first of June, the berries would be bitter. Belle gathered fresh herbs from the forest while she could, and began to prepare her medications. Small, tender raspberry leaves, slippery elm bark, mistletoe—good for clotting blood—squaw root, ginger, witch hazel and coltsfoot; all were abundant in the woods.

She then planted herb beds near the house for items she could not find in the woods. Marigold, garlic, cayenne pepper, turmeric, rosemary, horseradish and sage were some of her favorites to use for sickness. Belle increased the herbs she grew each year in her flowerbeds. She turned the soil in fall and added fertilizer, letting the ground rest for the spring planting.

She scrapped the pulp from a white willow, then dried it in the sun on a piece of screen and stored it in a Mason jar for future uses. The Native Americans had used white willow before the white man came to this area; it was the first aspirin. Comfrey—dried and ground into a pulp and mixed with petroleum jelly—made a good ointment for bruises. It aided in the healing of wounds or bones, and was also good for boils, rashes and psoriasis.

She gathered the dandelion roots and spread them out to dry in the sun. Then she chopped them into a mixture that could be brewed with water to make a tea taken internally. It was good for the liver, the gallbladder and blood pressure. Leaves of the dandelion made a good spring tonic when cooked, and when fried, it made an appetizing dish. She always kept her eyes open for the first sign of poke; it was a favorite food for Belle. A spring tonic, it was good eating when seasoned with bacon grease. She would gather as much as she could on her trips into the woods. If she found more than they could eat, she would can them for later use.

In the dark kitchen was a long table made from worn floorboards. Here, Belle mixed her herbs and prepared her breads for baking. Belle stored her herbs and tonics in Mason jars and covered baskets on shelves along the wall. In the old cupboard that had been her mother's, she kept herbs that needed to be stored in the dark. She kept many prepared tinctures and tonics, labeled and sealed in dark brown bottles. This helped keep the herbs from losing strength.

Belle tried to stay prepared at all times, never knowing when or what she might need. When the kitchen space was full, she stored her bitters in the cellar. They had built wooden shelves on one side of the interior walls in the cellar. The narrow pieces of shelving had a strip of wood placed halfway up in front of each shelf to keep the bottles from falling and shattering on the rock floor.

George started his job at the mines. He walked the three-mile trek each way. It was one of the best paying jobs in the area at $2 a day. Paydays were issued the first day of every month. On these days Belle would get herself dressed in her line-dried housedress, her feed sack apron and her high top canvas shoes. She then loaded her double-barreled shotgun and headed down the road with the gun on her shoulder, going to the mines to collect George's pay. It was a light moment for the other miners when they saw Belle coming down the road with the gun, but few messed with Belle, knowing that she could use the gun if she so chose.

The population of the Bickmore mining town increased daily as people moved into the area to work the mines. In fact, the population of Bickmore was greater than the county seat of Clay in the late 30s and 40s.

Crime increased and fights broke out as a variety of nationalities settled in. Chinese, Blacks, Italians and Irish, most good, hard-working people, but some liked to fight or drink and that made for trouble in the area. Some did not respect the tradition of other nationalities; some looked down upon those they did not understand. There seemed to be constant trouble as drinking men fought with knife or gun. Children who had lived this way all of their lives saw nothing wrong with intimidating the younger children.

Young Homer was attending a church service with his family at the Lilly School. He had several large scabs on his neck when some older boys behind him decided to tear the scabs off for him. He didn't say anything, knowing that his mother would not approve of it in church. But he made himself a promise that one day he would get the boy back who left his neck bleeding and burning. Later, when he was older and stronger, he met the boy at a pie social at school, walked up to him and, without warning, landed a fist in his nose, leaving the boy stunted and bleeding. Before he walked away he said, "That's for the time you tore scabs from my neck and made me bleed." The boy just looked on as he held his bleeding nose, but he never bothered Homer again.

FIGHTING WARTS

"It is going to be a hot day," Belle thought, as she was hoeing out the last row of her beans and corn. The sun had no mercy on her stooped back that had faced the sun since early morning. Her cotton dress was wet from sweating and the bonnet she wore to shield her face was damp and seemed to irritate her forehead. She lit into the last few stocks so she could get out of the sun. She hoped this would be the last hoeing to lay it over until harvest. She caught some movement out of the corner of her eye and she leaned on her hoe and looked that way. She saw a woman and four children walking up the road. The children followed the woman like a mother hen and her chicks. Belle finished the last of the hoeing and walked to the edge of the garden to wait for the people coming near. Belle was waving her apron in the wind to stir a breeze and cool her face. Hardly a leaf moved in the hot sun as she watched her company coming near.

"Howdy, Ms. Belle! I guess you don't remember me do ye?" the woman asked.

"Yell I know I have seen ye, but I don't recall your name," said Belle.

"I'm Goldie Ramsey. I live on Sycamore Creek and these are my youngins'. The least one is Bessie and that is why we come to see ye. Come here Bessie and let her see your elbow."

The little one came shyly and looked at the ground. Goldie took her arm and pushed up the sleeve of her sweater. Then she lifted her arm until Belle could see the wart on the little girl's elbow. It was raw and oozing beneath the large wart.

"That sure looks bad," said Belle as she took the arm and turned it some more, "how long has this been this way?"

"It's been getting worse for sometime now. I have used everything

I know and it just seems to get worse. So we decided to come today and let you look at it."

"Let me set down and cool off and I'll see what I can do. You all come to the porch and I'll get some cool water to drink."

They all walked over the foot log to the porch and found some chairs, while Belle was getting the water. She wet herself a towel and began to wipe the sweat and dirt from her face and hands. She took the water out and they sat just talking and cooling off. When they had rested, Belle had the little girl show her the arm again.

Belle said, "I can put some castor oil on it and it might make it drop off. You know, I don't profess to be a doctor; I mostly just deliver babies, but I can try to remove it. I rub the area around the wart and sometimes it works and sometime it don't."

Belle applied the castor oil and she then rubbed around the area and whispered a few words as she massaged the arm. Some said a spell might remove a wart. Belle didn't know but she would try it anyway.

"I'll give you a bottle of the oil and you apply it every day several times for about a week and then come back and let me take a look at it. Make sure it don't get infected, Goldie."

Belle went to get a small bottle and filled it with the oil from the castor bean that she had made last fall and took it to Goldie. They thanked her and headed off the hill for home.

After Belle cooled off from the hoeing she decided to go to the woods and look for some sassafras roots to make a good tea. She got her hoe and the cloth bag she carried on her shoulder and walked up the little holler past her house to look for the tree. It had a rough bark that was a light brown or gray; the tree grew twisted and had a rough scaly bark.

She had to look for a while before she came across the trees. She spotted some smaller ones beneath the tall one and she took the hoe and began to dig for the roots. She removed a lot of roots, shook the dirt away and placed them in the bag. She covered the exposed roots over again, to spare them until the next time.

She took time to look for some mushrooms while she was in the woods since it was near time for them. They usually grew beneath fruit trees or poplars. She had even found them along the creek.

It looked like the turkeys had been scratching in the dead leaves, so if there had been any mushrooms, the turkeys had destroyed them. Belle spotted and picked a few small morels, which were long on the stalk with small tops that looked like an umbrella. She walked back to the apple orchard down along the creek and stooped to look for some more. She was pleased to find several large yellow ones. She made several trips around the trees and failed to find anymore, but she planned to make a trip back here this week in search of more.

When she got back to the house she put the mushrooms in salt water and left them to soak. She dumped the sassafras roots out and took them to the branch running by her house. She swished them in the cold water until they were washed free of the dirt.

She then stripped the roots of their bark and sliced them with a sharp butcher knife. She put them in a large pot to simmer with some water. Soon the smell of sassafras invaded the house and porch. After it boiled for a while she would let it cool and then strain it to make a good drink. Native Americans of the area used the tea for painful joints, gastrointestinal problems, urinary track infections and profuse sweating to purge the body of impurities. The oil of the sassafras, called safrole, could be used to fight head lice, if used in small quantities. If taken internally it could be toxic. Some people have used it to purge the system of certain illnesses but it was not encouraged.

BELLE AND THE PAYCHECK

Belle was on one of her trips to the mines, walking down the road with her loaded shotgun on her shoulder. One of the mine owners was watching her from the window of the mining office. He asked the clerk at the office who the woman was who carried a loaded gun in every payday. He was told it was Mr. Neal's wife. "Okay, when she collects his pay today, tell Mr. Neal we won't be needing his services any longer." Belle's need to protect herself cost George a job.

BELLE FIGHTS NATURE

One hot sweltering day in late spring, the shrill sound of a whining horse broke the stillness of the little holler where Belle lived. She and George had just seated themselves on the little porch at their cabin to catch a cool breeze. As they looked up to the mountain road that wound steeply down to their home they spotted the silhouetted horse and rider against the sky. Belle arose and stood on her steps looking upward, knowing that the rider came for her! George leaned back on two legs of his cane-bottomed chair and whittled a whistle for the grandchildren as he watched the approaching rider.

At the sharp turn in the road near the foot of the mountain, the rider raised his hat to them as he neared the cabin. He brought the foaming horse to a stop at the foot-log by the house. Belle recognized Hiram Jones as he dismounted. He held the reigns of the prancing horse tight as he spoke to Belle.

"Granny, my woman will be needin' you soon."

Belle stood with her hands on her hips and said, "How far apart are her pains?"

"Getting close now," was his reply, "I was headin' for the second shift at the mines and she told me to alert you. Our oldest girl is tendin' to her now. Do you think you could go?"

"Yell, go on to work Hiram," she dismissed him with a fling of her hand, "I'll gather my things and be on my way. You done finished with your part anyway! How many youngun's this make you now, Hiram?"

"This will be the tenth. The twins are over two years old now," said a smiling Hiram.

"I'll get there in time to catch the new one, no doubt," said Belle as she went to get her medical bag. She entered the cabin, which was hot and dark—not even a breeze flowed inside—but she found her old black doctor's bag and checked the shelves for preparations she might need. From the rafters she snipped some dried corn silks and wrapped them in a small clean rag. She took a small brown jar of brewed mistletoe and placed it inside the bag. A new spool of black silk thread was placed in her apron pocket and then she grabbed a little brown bottle of sweet oil and added it to the bag. She added a change of clothes for herself and some clean rags. Lastly, she added a loaded gun to the doctor's bag.

Belle always went prepared for any unforeseen problems that could arise. She took the corn silk in case she had to make a poultice to stop hemorrhaging. A tea made from the corn silk and mistletoe would help the blood to clot. Black silk thread soaked in sweet oil was used for stitches. She worked quickly and efficiently, tucking a can of lard in one corner of the bag. She tucked some more clean rags around the items then zipped and buckled the bag.

She looked out the door and noticed the sky was quickly becoming overcast with rolling clouds. A breeze ruffled the leaves and the air smelled like rain. As she saddled her old nag, the storm began to move in and she could see flashes of lightning far off as the clouds rolled fast across the sky. She heaved her body up onto Old Boss and after a quick wave to George, she set out at a gallop, hoping that she could make it down Sycamore Creek before the rains swelled the creek crossings.

Old Boss's shod feet hit the damp ground with a thud. Belle never gave the horse any mercy as she switched her into a faster pace. Lightning flashed a threatening stream across the sky, closer now, and thunder cracked all around. Belle bent her body forward and tried to become as small as she could over the horse's head, as large balls of hail poured forth with a vengeance. Soon, Belle had to find shelter for herself and Boss. They could not tolerate much more of the hail. They finally entered a large stand of hemlock along the creek and took cover until the hail had passed. Belle took out her canvas coat with a hood and put it on. As she waited for the storm to subside, she thought with regret of the young tender plants in her garden, knowing that they would take a beating from the hail.

When the storm passed Belle set out to finish her journey. She led Old Boss to a large stump and mounted as the drizzle continued. Low clouds were hanging in the sky and the road was covered with balls of hail. Belle shivered as she came out onto the road and a rain-soaked breeze sent her to shaking. They continued on down the road. Not a soul showed their face as Belle and Old Boss tackled the muddy road and rising creek. As they neared a creek crossing, Old Boss was hesitant about entering the swollen water. She bucked and her eyes rolled as she stepped into the rushing water, but Belle was determined to cross, and with some nudging and switching, Boss started across.

The water was muddy and swift as the horse battled for a solid place to walk. Soon the swift water took control. It reached Belle's calves and proved to be cold, but Belle knew they had to get across. When they reached midstream, a nervous Old Boss began to swim. Belle draped herself low over the horse's neck and held on for dear life. They made it across, but the rushing water had carried them quite a distance downstream. Belle could see snakes swimming through the water; they apparently had been washed from their nests along the banks. She patted Boss to comfort her as they picked their way back to the road. Boss sensed danger and Belle held tightly to the reins as they made their way by the rushing water. All she needed now was snakebite!

Belle thought about how close she had come to losing a hold on the horse. If she had fallen off, there would have been no one to help her and she would have been long gone before anyone would know she was missing.

She reached the foot of the mountain and she could see the Walker family standing on their porch watching the storm and the rising creek. Belle saw a young girl standing at the corner of the house washing her hair in a barrel of rainwater. She just couldn't help but yell at her, "Fool girl! Don't you know that could kill you!"

The girl laughed and hollered back, "I do this every time it rains." Belle just shook her head and went "Huh!" as she rode away.

When Belle approached the two-story Victorian house that set back from the creek on a large flat bottom, she could see the children gathered on the porch. Some were sitting on chairs, some on the porch swing, and several on the banisters and steps. She called out a greeting and as she drew near, the children came rushing to meet her.

Peter, a boy of sixteen, came out and held the horse for Belle to get off. "Sure glad to see you Granny Woman. I was afraid you might not come because of the storm. Momma sure needs you though. We didn't know what to do, so we just kept looking for ye."

"Now son, no old storm could keep me away. Besides the Lord is looking out for me, I guess," she laughed. I guess He ain't ready to take me to heaven yet. Pete, you take care of Old Boss. Rub her down good and feed and water her. I owe her a lot."

"Yes Ma'am, I sure will," said Pete. "Go on in. Jo is with Mama. She'll be glad to see you."

Belle climbed the steps and rushed inside carrying her doctor's bag. One of the little ones was crying and Belle stopped to pat the little girl on the head and tell her that her Momma would be okay.

Belle found the room with the door shut and tapped lightly before entering. Jo was trying to help her mother but she looked scared to death. Belle had to wait for her eyes to adjust to the darkness of the room. She sat her doctor's bag down and opened it to remove items from within. "Jo, you go in and bring me a pan of hot water and another oil lamp. I need plenty of light."

"Sadie, I need to check and see how much the baby has crowned," she said, as Sadie was having another contraction. "Hold off bearing down, if you can, for a few more minutes." Belle removed two straps of leather from her doctor's bag. They were washed and ready for another delivery. She wrapped the ends around the footboard of the bed and buckled them tight. Then she handed the end that she had tied into a loop for handles to Sadie. "When you have the next pain, pull as hard as you can on these straps. Get ready now Sadie—it won't be long."

Belle continued to massage her belly, knowing she was in her hardest labor. "When I say 'push now' Sadie, you push." Sadie had not been able to talk but she listened to everything Belle had to say.

Belle took her place at the foot of the bed as Jo entered with the water and lamp. She put the lamp on a table near the foot of the bed for Belle. Belle dipped her hands in the warm water and then greased them with lard. As Sadie had another contraction, Belle placed her hands in the birth canal. She could feel that the baby had turned, so she placed both of her hands into the canal and turned the baby down headfirst. After another contraction, the baby's head emerged. "Doing good Sadie, just one or two more and I'll let you rest," said Belle as she watched the woman in labor.

"Here comes another one," yelled Sadie. "Alright, alright now, I am going to get up on the bed and help you push it out," said Belle. She climbed onto the foot of the bed and yelled, "now." Sadie gave one great heave and the baby slipped into Belle's waiting hands. She punctured the fluid sack that had protected the baby for nine months.

She turned the baby over and removed phlegm from the mouth. It was then that the baby gave its first cry into a new world. Belle placed it on its mother's stomach while she tied off the cord and cut it in two. "Looks like you got another fine girl, Sadie," Belle said as she wiped the baby off and wrapped it in a warm blanket that Jo had brought her. "Looks like I made it just in time for another youngin."

"We need to take care of the afterbirth now. You take this baby, Jo, and place her in that waiting basket. Sadie, I'm going to work the afterbirth down, so help me out."

Belle watched the afterbirth expel from the womb. She examined Sadie and saw that she would need a couple of stitches from tearing.

She removed the black silk thread, soaked it in sweet oil, then cleaned her hands with alcohol and sat about the task of stitching. Sadie hurt some, but Belle was persistent and soon had the stitches done. Belle placed clean, warm pads over and under Sadie and wrapped her in blankets. Belle examined the baby to see if all was well, then handed the new baby to its mother to feed while she buried the afterbirth.

When Belle came back inside, Jo had brought her a hot plate of food. Belle ate while the baby slept. "Sadie, that sure is a beautiful baby. What you goin' name this one?"

"I'm thinking I will name her after you, Belle—you have been so good to us. Rebecca Belle Jones—that sounds like it will do."

"That's good of you, Sadie; I ain't had many named for me! Have the youngin's been fed? I'll stay the night, though I think your girls can take care of everyone and Hiram will be home by then."

As darkness settled around the country home along the Sycamore Creek, the children were all in bed and the only sounds were those of rushing water and the rocking of the chair. Belle took the baby upon her shoulder and patted her to sleep as she rocked in a rocker on the porch. "Sleep little baby, for from this day forward you've got a heap of livin' to do." Crickets sang and peepers kept time in the darkness, Belle hummed a lullaby to the baby until she rocked the baby and herself to sleep. During the night Belle awakened and placed the baby in a bed made from a basket and placed it near the momma's bed. She returned to the porch and when she next awakened it was early morning.

Her old bones were stiff from yesterday's events and she had sat in the straight-back rocker most of the night, leaving her neck stiff. Belle went to check on her patients. Sadie had taken the crying baby to her breast so Belle puttered around, putting the room in order. She checked Sadie for hemorrhage and found she was doing fine. The aroma of fresh perked coffee and fried bacon flowed from the kitchen. Soon Jo brought Belle and Sadie a hot breakfast of bacon, eggs and biscuits, along with hot coffee. After finding her patients in good care and revived by a good hot meal, Belle went to saddle her horse.

Hiram came out on the porch as Belle was leaving, "I can't pay you much Granny Woman, but I have a couple pieces of silver I been holdin' back for ye," he said, as he walked toward Belle and handed her the money.

"Well, I thank ye, Hiram. I would have come anyway, but I surely do appreciate the money. Take care of the baby and Sadie. I hope you won't need me again too soon!" said Belle with a laugh as she headed up the creek toward home.

She was nearing Charlie's Fork, where the creek had broken over into the road. She had to guide Old Boss carefully over the sharp stones and the bed of slimy rocks and mud. The horse stopped to take a drink and Belle sat patiently looking out over the woods. When she spotted a few sprouts of raspberry vine near the creek, she got down and picked a few, wrapped them in a clean rag, and placed them in her apron pocket. She would take them home and crush them to make a tonic, which would alleviate morning sickness. Women in the community frequently asked Belle what to do for morning sickness. Few women had time to slow down with it, as their large families still required their care.

Boss snorted as she finished her drink and waited for Belle. Belle and Boss slowly started the climb up the ridge toward home.

When they reached the crossroads on top of Beechy, Old Boss didn't need any coaxing from Belle. She just held on as Boss hurried down the road toward home. Boss knew that a warm barn and feed was just ahead.

WASH DAY

As they came around the turn in the road, Belle had a full view of her home and saw that there was smoke coming from the chimney. She knew that Radar would be fixing a good meal. After Belle ate a hot meal of navy beans, hot cornbread with butter and wilted lettuce salad, she lay down on her bed to rest for a while and soon dozed off to sleep.

When she awakened she began to gather the clothes that needed washing. She went on the hunt for her big copper kettle and took it down by the branch that ran close to the house. Radar had started a fire for her and she hauled water to the kettle with two 5-gallon buckets. While she waited for the water to heat, she sliced pieces from the lye soap she made and added it to the water. Taking the washboard, she began with the white clothes. She stripped the sheets from the beds and then added the towels. She stirred the pot and added a little bluing. When these were washed and wrung by hand, she took them to the running stream and dashed them in the water until the suds were gone. Then she wrung them again and put them out to dry on bushes and on clothes lines. Next she washed the dark clothes and heavy pants and dresses. She scrubbed until her knuckles were raw and then she hung the remaining items on the lines. She dragged the copper tub to the porch and scrubbed the floor with the water, then turned the kettle over to dry and hung her mop and broom up on nails on the porch.

Feeling that she had done enough for an old woman for one day, she sat down on her freshly scrubbed porch and enjoyed a cup of coffee.

DISASTER STRIKES

Belle went to the post office one morning and heard that a fire had raged through a house at Red Row. It had taken three little children and left two burned badly. The mother had gone out and left the children alone. That infuriated Belle and she said that a woman who goes out running around at night did not need children.

As soon as Belle got her mail she walked on down to the location of the burned house and asked about the children. Someone directed her to a house where the children had been taken; she went to see if she could help. Belle had seen many people injured or hurt in some way, but this nearly broke her heart. She looked down on the little children—a girl of about four and a boy near 12. The story goes that one of the children started a fire in the fireplace and caught their clothes in the flame. The house was old and the wood burned easy. As the children tried to put the fire out, they too were burned. Finally when they could do no more, the 12 year old gathered the little girl in his arms and ran, thinking the others were behind him. When he discovered they were still inside, it was too late to go back in.

Belle examined the children and shook her head. She knew that their need was far beyond what she could do, but she sat down between the beds they lay on and prayed for them. A patient burned this badly was something she did not know how to care for and it grieved her to see the agony the children were in. The little girl passed away the following day; the boy lasted two more days. The people in the community had taken on the responsibility of the forsaken children. They buried them all on the same day. It was a tragedy that hit home for everyone who heard it. The mother left the area and everyone thought it was best she did, for her pain would be remembering how her children had died.

GOIN' FOR A VISIT

One day in July, Belle decided to visit her niece Marilda and see how the family and the new baby were doing. It wasn't a difficult walk to the Osborne's. They just lived over the hill from Belle. Belle set out at mid-morning and stopped along the way to talk with neighbors. She especially wanted to stop at Marv and Lou Brown's to see how her grandchildren were doing. She ran into Homer and Forest heading home after they had picked huckleberries. They were carrying a large tub between them that was full, and each carried a bark basket on their back that was also full. "Looks like a good year for berries this year, boys," said Belle.

"Yell, they are thick this year," said Forest.

"Mommy told us to pick as many as we could find," said Homer, "she likes to put up a lot for winter."

"We been a pickin' since daybreak," said Forest.

Belle and they boys walked down the mountain path toward home. When they arrived, Marilda was washing Mason jars for the berries and baby Ann was asleep on the front room bed. Ruth was cooking supper and John and Clem were outside playing. Bib was at the mines.

"Hello, Aunt Belle," said Marlida, as she saw the trio coming up the walk, "ain't seen you for awhile. How you been?"

"Oh, I been alright for an old woman, I guess. I been busy though, delivering babies. Can't even get my garden worked up. I guess it's a good thing we got Radar. I just wanted to see how the baby was doing."

"She's doing right well. I put her down a while ago, so she'll be awake soon and you can carry her around for a while. Deretha had another girl, didn't she?"

"Yell, I need to stop and see to her and the baby, born the last of June. They called her Cordelia Belle, after me and Dilly."

Just then Clem and John came running in, wanting a cold biscuit to last them until suppertime. Belle swatted their little butts and teased them until they had fixed their biscuits with blackberry jam.

John turned around as he left and said, "When Poppy comes home he'll call me little Johnny Hunk." They all laughed at that. Ruth was mad because the boys had left a mess on the table that she had just cleaned.

"I guess you know we are having a revival at the schoolhouse, Belle," said Marilda.

"Yell, I'm plannin' on goin' if I don't have to walk that distance in the dark. What night you and Dilly goin'?"

"It starts on Sunday night. If you want to ride with us, come down and leave with us: Poppy is goin' take us in the wagon."

"I'll be here then," said Belle. Just then baby Ann awoke and Belle went to pick her up and juggle her on her knee.

Marilda continued to wash jars and clean huckleberries as she talked to Belle. "Why don't you take enough of these berries to make a cobbler, Belle?"

"Yell, I'd like that a heap, Rildy. I'll get Radar to make one; he's a better cook than me anyway."

Marilda took a cardboard box and placed some huckleberries in the bottom and covered them with a clean cloth. After Belle had visited awhile, she said she would leave and check on Deretha and the new baby. She thanked Marilda for the berries and headed up the road to visit with Okey and Deretha.

On the night of the revival Belle cleaned herself up and put on a fresh dress. She loaded her shotgun and carried a lantern as she walked down the mountain path toward her niece's home. When she arrived, they were trying to get everyone together. John brought his wagon around; he had loaded it with bales of hay. Marilda took several blankets and spread them across the hay. The children crawled in along with Belle and Marilda while Dilly rode in the front.

When they got to the schoolhouse, people were already swarming around. The kids jumped out and headed out to play. The women walked to the school. John unhitched his horses and took them to the creek to drink. The preacher welcomed them to the service and Vernon Neal led the singing. Brother Vernon was married to Leslie, one of Dilly's girls. The desks had been pushed against the wall and the center was bare except for the potbellied stove. Most people just stood around the outside walls or sat on the desks. They could hear the men who stayed outside talking in low voices, since the windows had been left up for a cool breeze.

That meeting sparked one of Bickmore's greatest revivals of the decade. The more the preacher spoke of hell's fire and damnation, the more the people shouted and sang. Many nights, people living along the road would hear Belle and her sisters, Dilly and Marilda, heading home by wagon, still full of the spirit. People poured into the little schoolhouse to attend the revival they had heard so much about. Many souls were renewed and there were many new converts.

It was quiet in the holler as they went back to Marilda's. Belle went in the house to get her shotgun and lantern. The family could hear her as she walked toward home with the loaded shotgun on her shoulder and a swinging lantern burning bright in her hand. She was singing *Amazing Grace* as she climbed the mountain trail toward home.

A TIME TO HARVEST

Belle stepped out from her porch to look at the colorful hills and feel the fresh air of a new fall. It was her favorite time of year because it was so peaceful and the bounty of the harvest was ready to gather. The sunshine falling on the rustling leaves of every color seemed to give her old body more pep, while the gentle breeze of autumn satisfied her soul. She knew that winter was coming and she wanted to make the most of the days before the cold.

She went out to her herb garden and removed the bloom, the seed, and the leaves from her plants. She cleaned the flowerbeds and checked on the pens of geese and chickens and her horse and cow. She made a mental note to repair the wire on the chicken pens. She walked across the road from her house to look at the last of the garden. She checked and there seemed to be several big pumpkins and some Kershaw (white pumpkin). It made a better pie than the yellow. She stopped to examine the late heads of cabbage and decided to check the signs for pickling. She would gather those left and make a crock of sauerkraut for winter.

She walked up to the little orchard along the creek and picked up a few of the last apples. She examined the tree of winter pears and when the frost hit, she would come and gather the load and store it in the cellar. She looked for some wild grapes and found them growing on the side of the mountain near the garden. She picked them and carried them home in her apron. She cleaned them and cooked them and made them into jelly.

Birds were flying south and they made a continuous racket as they flew over the mountains in swarms. Belle was wondering just where the summer went. It seemed that only yesterday she was planning her spring garden. It had been a good year for vegetables and with the cellar loaded for winter, she wondered if the winter would be a rough one. She had to stay close to home when it was cold and the days seemed to drag. Only a true emergency would determine if she would go out.

George liked the winter. He sat by the fireplace and whittled out walking sticks and whistles. Belle and George both liked to chew their tobacco and once in a while they smoked their pipes. When George grew tired he would lean back in his mule-eared chair and doze. Radar preferred to be alone and he cooked and rambled around the farm. Belle's nature was to get things done as quickly as she could, and it tired people to watch her as she worked.

Belle still kept a milk cow and she went everyday to milk, churning when needed. She walked out to the shed and spent some time with Old Boss. She brought her handfuls of fresh greens and an apple now and then. The old horse was too old to keep up a schedule of carrying humans, but Belle could not see killing the horse. Besides, if the horse had not been with her, she would have died with some of the things she encountered on her rides to doctor.

Winter hit early. It swept down one day without warning; brushing the limbs of the trees and the sprouts of grass with a new white coat of snow. Trees that had not shed their leaves cracked like the shot of a gun as they broke from the heavy snow.

The cold winds blew through the cracks of the cabin and slipped in beneath the doors. Belle stuffed some rags into the cracks in the windows and she made a long narrow rope of scraps of material and stuffed it with rice so she could lay them in front of the doors to keep the cold out. She started working on some rag rugs and she made them big enough to cover almost the entire floor of the living area and kitchen.

They kept a healthy fire in the fireplace and in the kitchen stove. Belle would cook more when she was snowed in than she did in the summer months.

She thought about making some spicy pumpkin pies and loaves of pumpkin bread. She got a little bowl and a bag of walnuts and sat down in front of the fire. She began cracking the nuts and placing them in the bowl, stopping to eat a piece of the walnuts now and then. She got the nuts cracked and got out the bowls, the flour, the spices, shortening, sugar and eggs. She made piecrust for four pies, stoked the fire and greased the pans. Then she made the filling with the eggs, milk and sugar. She had to beat them hard to make the filling smooth. She slipped the pies into the oven and checked the time.

While they were baking, she used the leftover pumpkin and stirred up two pans of pumpkin bread. She added the walnuts, eggs, sugar, spices and flour; she lined her pans with shortening and covered them until the oven was empty. The aroma of the pumpkin pies floated about the house and soon Radar and George wondered when the pies would be ready. Belle told them the pies would have to cool, but when the bread was done she would slice it in thick slices and make some fresh coffee; they could have that first.

Belle removed the pies and set them on the table to cool. She placed the loaves in the oven and when she thought they were near done, she perked a pot of coffee. While she waited for both, she sat near the fireplace in her rocker and read from her Bible.

It was hard to do the laundry in the winter months, but they had no choice. Belle always brought her tubs into the house and heated the water on the cook stove. She would sort the colors and wash the white items first by scrubbing each on the washboard. Then she would rinse them in the other tub, wring them by hand and take them to her porch and hang them to dry. Sometimes it would take awhile to dry them and she would have to bring them inside and finish drying them in front of the heat.

She washed the dark heavy clothes and hung them on the porch. She tried not to wash blankets and bedding in winter if she could help it, because it was so messy and hard to wring things out. She poured hot water into a wash pan and added some lye soap. Then she soaked her kitchen towels and stirred the water with a wooden paddle. She doused them in clean rinse water and wrung them out to dry. She would hang them near the cook stove on wire hangers with clothespins. Belle thought she might like winter weather better if such ordinary things as laundry did not create such hard work.

Belle, her family and her neighbors all worked hard in the fall to be prepared for a long cold winter. If they did not prepare, it could mean death and starvation. There was no time for being lazy in the isolated areas of Clay County in the 1920s and 30s. Every neighbor was willing to help someone who was helping themselves; some butchered hogs and beef. If others were willing to come and share the load of butchering, they would go home with a portion of the meat.

If someone had a large orchard and did not need all of the fruits, they traded that for some firewood or coal. The neighbors all around helped one another, because they each knew that it meant survival for all. People in the mountains knew what was expected of them and they depended on each other to live. If someone fell ill and they needed a doctor, they could get Belle to tend the patient. Instead of money, they could give Belle a sack of fresh ground cornmeal or some feed for her animals. If she needed a load of firewood, she would trade canned goods or doctoring.

The rhythm of the mountain people always ran smooth as long as both sides kept their word. If there was a feud among families, then the other neighbors tried to stay neutral. The habit of clan living was brought from Ireland, Scotland, Italy and England. When checking family trees it is evident that people here in the mountains never went far to marry, probably due to the hardships of traveling. Trails or paths were their routes of travel and these had to be maintained by the owners of the land. Few real public roads were constructed. Most of the ways of travel were horse, sled or walking. Some could spend their entire life never traveling more than twenty miles from home.

SOME ARE BORN AND SOME DIE

In late August 1937, Belle and George were sitting on their porch in the evening trying to catch a cool breeze. The day had been one of record heat and it didn't help the house any that Belle and Radar had been canning tomatoes all day. George was sitting on his mules-ear-tobacco chair with two legs on the floor, leaning against the wall, and he was whittling. Belle was sitting on the steps with a wet cloth, wiping her face and arms. All was quiet in their little haven and in the stillness they heard the gallop of a horse. They looked to the sharp turn in their road and soon spotted a horse and rider. Belle knew that she was needed somewhere. When the man drew up near the front steps, Belle noticed he was a stranger.

"Granny Woman, could you come to attend a birth? It's my daughter and there seems to be a problem."

"I'll get my things. George, saddle my horse," said Belle as she hurried to gather her supplies. She was ready in record time and the man waited impatiently atop the horse, neither he nor George tried to have a conversation. When George led Old Boss out of the stable, he helped heave Belle up and they set off down the road. It was nearing twilight and it was hard to see what was ahead, but the man kept going and Belle kept close behind.

They went down the creek, then turned up Middle Creek until they reached the road that led up to Leatherwood. When they neared the top, the man stopped long enough for Belle to catch up. Then he pointed to a narrow path on his left. She followed him along the trail. Brush swept out every now and then and scratched Belle on the arms and legs; she ignored it and followed the man in.

They soon stopped along the path where the trail dipped down into a bowl. Belle could see a small house and the weak flame from a kerosene light.

"This way," the man said, nearing the house.

"You go on in and I'll take care of the horse," he said.

Belle untied her satchel from the saddle and, without a word, went quickly up the steps. When she neared the door, she could hear a woman crying. She found the patient upon a bed in the corner and another woman, whom Belle assumed was the mother, patting her and trying to console her.

The woman turned as Belle sat her bag down. "We sure are glad to see you, Granny. I don't know what else to do; the baby just won't come and she's been this way now for many hours."

"Just move over and let me take a look; bring that lamp a little closer. There now, girl, I am here to help you; this will soon be over. Bring me some warm water, woman, and some fresh linens." Belle washed her hands in the pan of water and then greased them from a can of lard she kept in her supplies.

"Little girl, I am going to turn this baby and you have to help me. It's goin' to pain you, but we have to do it, so listen to my voice and do the best you can."

The exhausted girl looked to be about sixteen and scared to death, but she readily agreed to help Belle.

Belle slid her greased hands into the birth canal and felt a shoulder lodged there. She found the head and when the girl had another pain, Belle turned the baby's head down.

"Okay now girl, let's get this little one out. When one more pain comes along, you push when I say push. Mother, get over here and push on the stomach when I tell you to." She motioned to the woman standing in the corner with her hands over her mouth and a worried look on her face.

"Okay, here we go. PUSH, PUSH! Here it comes." Belle caught the baby as it shot into the world. The cord was wrapped twice around the child's neck. She removed it quickly. Without a word she cleaned the baby's mouth and tapped its toes to revive it. She worked with the baby to no avail. Belle then laid the little girl upon her mama's stomach while she cut the cord and tied it off. The baby was very blue and the girl's mother said, "Why is the baby not crying?"

The girl began to get upset. Belle cleaned the little baby and wrapped it in a piece of sheeting, then handed it to the girl.

"It didn't make it, little girl; I'm sorry. The labor was too long and it strangled hours ago. You take a while and hold the baby while I take care of you. She sure is a beautiful baby."

The mother and daughter both cried silently as they held the baby for the first and last time. Belle cleaned the girl up, adding fresh linens beneath her and placing warm pads between her legs to stop the bleeding after she had expelled the afterbirth. Then she took the afterbirth to the father, who was waiting on the porch. "You take this and bury it, and then you can come in."

He took the bucket without a word and walked toward the woods. Belle went back inside and asked the girl if they had any clothes to dress the baby in for burial.

The older woman said that they had not prepared for the birth because she and the father did not know the girl was expecting until she went into labor. Belle asked her to find some scraps of material and she would make a little gown for the baby. When the father returned and came into the room, he looked down upon his daughter and the newborn baby. His behavior showed much disapproval, but he didn't say a word to the girl.

While Belle sat in the rocker sewing the little gown, she asked the man if he had a box in the barn that could be used for the baby's coffin. He said he would get something and bring it in. Belle stitched the little white gown, made of flannel. She found a scrap of green ribbon and made two little flowers at the neck. She then went to the girl and said, "It's time now, honey. I need to have the baby so I can clean her up and put this dress on her. Have you decided on a name?"

"I don't know any; do you, Momma?" The girl asked as tears rolled down her cheeks.

"We can name her Sarah after my mother, if you want to."

"Yes, I would like to name her Sarah," the girl said.

Belle took the baby, and as the women watched, she cleaned the baby's little blue body with sweet oil and then dressed her in the little gown she had made. "Would you like a piece of her hair to keep?" Belle asked the girl.

"Oh yes, could I?" asked the girl. "Well, I don't see why not, she's yours, ain't she?" Belle said, as she took her scissors and snipped a little tuft of dark hair from the baby's head and handed it to the mother. "Put this in a piece of paper and keep it for a memory."

The man brought in a little wooden crate and Belle lined it with an old sheet. Then she went to the girl and said, "Honey, it's time now to lay the baby in her bed."

The girl was reluctant to give the baby up, but knew she must. She took one last look at the chubby little face, the head of dark hair, and the little hands and feet, all so perfectly formed. She kissed the little head and handed her to Belle. Without another word, Belle placed the baby in the box and the man started to place the lid on and nail it shut. "Wait until you get outside to do that," said Belle, "I'll stay here with the girl, and you and your woman can find a place for burial. Go on now."

They left and Belle sat by the grieving daughter until she went to sleep. Then Belle dozed, too.

When the first rays of sun shone through a side window, Belle aroused herself with a shake and a hand over her face. The woman brought her some hot coffee. She drank until the cup was empty and the man had brought her horse to the front steps. She took one last look at the sleeping girl and grieved for her, knowing she would never forget her loss.

The woman thanked her for coming as she mounted from the porch steps. The man led the way out and Belle followed. When they reached the road, he paused and turned to talk to Belle. "Granny Woman, I thank you for coming. I ain't got much money, but I have been saving these two silver dollars for sometime. I guess this is a good time to spend them. We didn't know the girl was expectin'. She hadn't been away from the house so we were shocked."

"Mister, you don't have to give the money to me. Go on and save them some more. As for the girl and the baby, you know these things happen. Just be glad we saved the girl. Don't be too hard on her now—losing the child was punishment enough."

"No, I want you to have these coins," he said and handed them to Belle.

"I thank you kindly. I didn't catch your name," said Belle.

"I didn't offer it, either," said the man, "It's best we leave it at that."

As Belle rode on down the road, she turned and looked back but no one was there. The man had already disappeared into the woods. She shuddered, shook her head, and wondered if this had all been a dream!

A HELPING HAND

Belle received word from the schoolteacher at Bickmore School that a Chinese family had moved into the coal camp. The son, who attended school, said that his mother was expecting a baby, did not speak English and did not know who to ask for help. Belle found out where she lived and went to visit when the son was there to speak for his mother.

Belle could see that they were poorer than most and alienated by others in the coal camp. She felt sorry for the woman and kids. The father moved them wherever he could get work and that was the best they could do. Belle asked some questions and told the woman she would come back when her delivery date was near.

About three weeks had passed when she returned to the house. It was a pitiful sight—hardly any food, no furniture and very little clothing. The condition of the home was a shambles. Water had to be carried from the community well that was a half-mile away. Belle brought some food to fix while she was there and also cleaned up the house. She scrubbed and cleaned and cooked a hot meal for the family. She could see the appreciation on the woman's face.

She told the children stories, and sometimes the oldest son had to interpret for the others. She knew these children had a bleak future ahead of them and she wanted to give them some kindness while she could. She held the baby girl of two on her lap and rocked her to sleep. The other children spread a ragged blanket on the floor and Belle had no choice but to place the sleeping baby there. The mother lay on a lumpy mattress on an old iron bed. The children all slept on the floor. Belle had brought herself a quilt and pillow, but she gave them to the children and slept sitting up on a wooden chair.

As Belle road her horse up Route 16 the next day, she took in the scenes of coal camp living. It was a depressing sight, but at least those who lived and worked here had enough to eat and a roof over their head. When Belle got close to the houses they called Rock Cut, she looked over at a house and noticed a woman standing out in her yard. She was looking up at the sky and talking to herself. Belle thought that was a strange thing to do and she rode over to the woman's house and asked her if everything was all right. The woman had her back to Belle but when she turned around, Belle could see a bewildered look on her face. She was dressed in ragged clothes and her hair was long and standing on end. Her face was smeared with ashes and her feet were bare.

She didn't say much, but Belle got down off the horse and walked toward her, asking again, "Is everything all right here?"

The woman continued to look up to the sky and she said, "No one ever comes to visit anymore, and I just get so lonesome that I come outside and talk to God. My man was killed in the mines here, and my children grew up and moved away. I ain't much good to anyone anymore."

Belle could see that she was a little confused but knew that she was mostly just lonesome. "Well, I think I would like to stay and visit with you today. Do you have any coffee? I could use a cup."

The woman was so pleased to have company that she raced right in her house and made some coffee. They sat down on the porch and Belle learned a lot about the woman. She was the one people called "Crazy Carolyn." But what they didn't know was that Carolyn wasn't near as crazy as some who called her that. She was confused and lonesome, and Belle was going to make it a point to stop and visit when she was going by. She mounted the horse, but turned to wave at a now-smiling Carolyn.

GATHERING HERBS FROM THE MASTER'S STORE

In late September, Belle decided to take a day to gather herbs, or 'bitters' as they were called in the mountains. She draped a gunnysack, with a strap she had sewn on, over her shoulder. She got a roll of clean rags and placed them in her apron pocket, went to fetch her 'sang' hoe, put on some long heavy socks that covered her legs up to her knees and headed for the woods. She followed a stream that would take her to the cherry orchard on top of the mountain.

The forest was alive with trees of yellows and reds as the leaves began to turn. A carpet of crisp leaves covered the ground, and a warm breeze sent forth an aroma of clean fall air. As she walked along she kept her eyes peeled for plants she needed.

She first came upon several large clumps of mullein. These leaves, when made into a poultice, would stop hemorrhaging from the bowels and improved the lungs when taken internally. The leaves were made into a tea and used to help asthmatics. A poultice from the leaves could stop swelling of a stiff neck and sore muscles. She would crush the flowers and steep them in oil, which made a good ointment for bruises and frostbite. Bruised leaves could be used for diaper rash, although Belle preferred a spoon of raw cornmeal.

Belle gathered the large clumps and shook them free of dirt. She wrapped them in a clean rag and placed them at the bottom of the sack. She kept walking up the mountain, following the gurgling branch. She kept her eyes peeled for some goldenseal or yellow root, knowing that she had gathered it here before. When she recognized the leaves of the plant, she removed her bag and began to dig the root. When she had a sizable amount of the root, she wrapped it in a rag and tied it with a string. She never took more of any of the plants then she could use—that was the rule of the wilderness.

She would spread the roots on a screen to dry, and then grind them into a powder made into a tincture. This could be taken internally for sluggish digestion. She would make a concoction by cutting the roots into small pieces and boiling it for about 30 minutes. Then she would strain it and store it in clean brown bottles, and place in her cellar until she would need it. It could be used for many different aliments: head colds, mouth infections, skin conditions, digestion, stomach cramps.

Belle made it to the top of the mountain where she had to sit down and rest. Climbing up mountain paths was harder for Belle these days. She did not move as fast as she once had, and it took her longer to recover from a day of hard work. Everything was quiet and peaceful here in the orchard; she closed her eyes and leaned back to rest on the trunk of a tree. She felt the breeze blowing softly across her face, ruffling her hair as it blew by. She could hear the rustling sound of the bird's feet as they hunted for food in the crisp leaves. Not a sound could she hear except for those of nature. The world was far away when Belle was gathering herbs.

She was in the cherry orchard looking for some cherry bark to use in cough syrups. When she found the tree she wanted to use, she removed a large knife from her apron pocket and sliced through the bark. She wrapped it and placed it in her sack.

She knew that a patch of ginseng grew nearby, so she hunted until she found it. She removed the roots from the ground with her hoe, shook the excess dirt off and discovered that she had several three prong roots. After she wrapped the roots, she took the berries and replanted them for future use. Ginseng was a prized item to the mountain people. It sometimes meant cash money for those who had very little. It could be sold at a local store first, and then purchased by China to use for medicinal purposes. But it was also a necessity for those who could not afford or get to a doctor. Belle knew that ginseng was a valuable herb and could be used for many aliments. It would strengthen the immune system, gave energy, and was good for mental stimulation and emotional and physical well-being. Belle would dry the ginseng on frames of screen and then seal it in a Mason jar and label it for future use.

Evening was casting shadows along the mountain and Belle thought she would head down the hill for home. She followed the mountain stream and was careful where she stepped; she used her hoe for a walking stick. When she reached a little waterfall along the creek, she removed her heavy sack from her shoulder and cupped her hands for a refreshing drink of cold mountain water. It was a peaceful setting, with no one around to penetrate the blissful stillness; the only sound was of her own breathing and the birds singing in the trees. After she had rested for a while, she started down the mountain. She knew that witch hazel grew close to the creeks and she kept her eye out for a tree. Near the bottomland, where they had an apple orchard, Belle spotted a witch hazel tree. The tree was easy to recognize. It was usually of small stature, grew near a water source and had a small spike at the base of the leaves.

Upon crushing the leaves, they had a distinct, refreshing smell. Belle gathered some of the leaves and laid them flat on a clean rag. She rolled it up, tied it to keep the leaves from being crushed, and carefully placed the package into her apron pocket. The bark was also used to make tinctures or salves, which could be used for skin problems or soaked on pads and laid over the eye. It could be taken internally for diarrhea and used as a healing ointment to fight inflammation. It could be mixed with petroleum jelly to keep the wounds from drying out. She scraped the bark and shred the internal part of the tree to use for infusions. She spotted a water birch and went to cut a few of the smaller branches. She wrapped them in an airtight bag. She liked to cut the end of a birch and fan it out to use for cleaning teeth. The chewed bark left a refreshing taste in the mouth. When she had packed the witch hazel and birch, she started for home.

When she got to the house, she removed each item and washed it well in the cold water of the creek running by her house. She dried the water from the herbs and laid them out to air dry in the sun; some she tied with twine and hung them from the porch rafters. When they were dried to her satisfaction, she sealed and stored them, never knowing when she might need them.

Belle and George both used tobacco and when they finished a

pack, they folded the wrappers and placed them around their fireplace mantle, or the fireboard as Belle called it, until it was full. They hung small wind chimes from their ceiling and when the breeze blew through the open door, the sound of many wind chimes soothed the soul. Belle and George were eccentric, but maybe that is what kept them a couple for all their years together.

In October, Marilda, Belle and Leslie liked to set a day aside to make apple butter. They put all the apples they could harvest together. They set a large copper kettle in the yard at Marilda's, and the kids cut and stacked firewood. On the first day, they peeled the apples and cooked it into applesauce. The following day, they added the spices and sugar to sweeten the sauce. Marilda always liked to pour a bag of cinnamon candies in for flavor.

Everyone in the families stopped by to visit or to take a turn at stirring. It had to be stirred constantly to keep the sauce from sticking to the bottom of the kettle and ruining the whole batch. The workers collected some coins of copper and silver and washed them until they gleamed. These were put into the kettle to keep the sauce from sticking to the bottom. Someone always kept the fire going and watched the flames, never letting them get too high. Smoke from the fire clung to their clothing and hair, but the scent of cinnamon made their mouths water. Their backs were tired from stirring and their hands were calloused from the stirring paddle. Others took a turn at washing canning jars, and still others fixed a picnic for the workers. By the end of the second day, everyone was weary and glad the job was finished. They packed the apple butter into sanitized jars and sealed the tops. Then they divided the lot among the workers, to be stored in their cellars until winter.

PREPARING FOR OLD MAN WINTER

In the fall, Belle and George began harvesting their crops and gathering nuts and fruits to store for the long winter. As fall mornings became cooler, they butchered a hog and hung it in the smokehouse. Getting up in years, neither George nor Belle was able to cut and stack firewood, their main source of heat.

When they found someone who sold bituminous coal, they started using that for heat and cooking. They had to find someone with a truck to go and get their coal. They found a man, Mr. Stone, in Lizemore, whom they liked to purchase coal from; he always gave them more for their money. The coal burned with a smoky yellow flame and was not as pleasant as wood, but it was easier to obtain. Belle asked her nephew Homer to take his truck and bring her a load of coal. Belle had always been so good to Homer and all of his brothers and sisters that he was glad to help her.

During the winter months, the sulfur smell and the sight of smoke from the chimneys, hanging low in the sky due to the barometric pressure, could be a depressing site in the mountains. But the people who lived in these mountains had to do whatever it took to survive Mother Nature's fierce winter.

They, like their ancestors of Welsh, Irish and Scottish descent, learned to survive, no matter how hard the conditions. Their predecessors came to settle this land and continued to move deeper into the mountains and farther away from society. That isolation cost them dearly, for they struggled to maintain a small farm on a steep side of poor land, much more suited to hunting than farming. But when they came, they stayed, and their children and grandchildren knew no other way of life. The stories of their ancestors were told and retold to each generation in the oral tradition, as many of the older generation did not read or write. Ballads telling of death and sadness were memorized and sung when they gathered for a party or wedding or even at a death. Young children learned to play the string instruments that had been brought from across the water, in turn keeping the history of their people alive from one generation to the next.

Their traditions, the way they worshipped and the words that integrated their language—even their pronunciation of words—were mostly preserved. Maybe two generations before, they had called themselves Irish or Scot, but now they were called mountaineers, and most of the time, their neighbors were relatives. They spoke their Elizabethan English and stayed bound together, just as clans had done in the old country.

Maybe it was tradition or maybe it was out of necessity, but they never traveled far from their roots. They acquired large plots of land deep in the wilderness that others did not want. Here they built their homes and sub-divided their lands as their children married and began families of their own. They scratched out a living and raised their young and the land was divided again and again.

When their time came to go, they knew they would be buried near home and they, too, would become a permanent piece of this land. Today, small forgotten cemeteries dot the landscape. When wandering deep into the mountains, one may stumble upon an old graveyard marked with fieldstones for headstones. Only those others who had also passed on would have known the names. While looking around you may identify the remains of a cabin, a spring, or flowers that faithfully bloom, even when no one is there to attend them. Stop and listen! You may hear a mother calling her children home, or, off in the distance, the faint sounds of laughter. The memories are all that's left of a pioneer family that has now vanished.

HIGH ON A MOUNTAIN

A storm was brewing one evening, with lightning flashing and thunder crashing all about. George and Belle had retired early. Belle was just dozing off when she thought she heard a knock on the door. She got up to check and reached for her shotgun by the door. She held a candle in her left hand and looked out into the face of a young stranger. Belle waited for him to speak. "Sorry to disturb you, Granny, but I didn't know who else to ask. I have a friend who lives way back on the mountain. I went there today to check on him, and he is sick with a fever and out of his head. Do you think you could make the trip to see him?"

She talked low so as not to awaken George and Radar, "Come in and wait by the door here; I'll get ready."

She pulled her doctor's bag out from beneath her bed and set it on the table to check her supplies. She added some teas she thought she might need, some camphor, some mullein and a piece of flannel. She slipped her loaded handgun inside and went to dress for the wet weather. She pulled on a pair of George's long underwear and then her dress and apron. She found a pair of old rubber boots and put them on over her canvas shoes. She then donned a waterproof shawl and looked around to see if she would need anything else. She looked over at the man and with a nod she was ready to go. The man seemed very anxious to be on his way. He reached for her bag and carried the lantern as she fell in line behind him. She could see his old battered car ahead. It was rusted and held together in places with wire. He had to turn the key several times before the engine finally turned over.

They started down toward Sycamore on a rough road, rattling and slipping in the deep ruts. There was no glass in the windows and spatters of rain blew in. Belle held on and didn't say much. She was worried that the creek crossings would drown out the engine of the car, but they made it through. They parked the car on higher ground above the creek and started walking.

The man said, "Granny, I hated to bring you out here tonight, but I'm not sure my friend would make it another day if I didn't get help. He seems to have been sick for several days. I just decided to stop for a visit and found him out of his head and tossing and turning on his bed."

They resumed their walk through a dense, covered path that climbed to a steeper incline as they went along. They finally reached a small plateau and stopped to catch their breath. The thunder and lightning still rumbled in the distance. The rain had stopped, but the trees and bushes dripped water everywhere.

The man said, "This last part of the climb is more dangerous in the dark. I'll carry your bag and you take the lantern. I'll go first and you stay close behind me. One wrong step and you could roll to the bottom of this rock cliff. Hug the wall and watch your step; I'll lead you on."

As they continued around the ledge, Belle could hear dogs barking in the distance. "I guess those old hounds can smell us coming," Belle thought, as they inched along the narrow path. They reached a narrow mountain stream that was rushing down the hill. The man jumped across and raised his voice over the water as he coached her across. He held out his hand and Belle stepped into the stream. She was a little unstable on her feet, but the hand of the young man reached out to grasp hers, and pulled her onto the path.

They climbed another small incline and parted the dense hemlock to find a path. Now they were looking up and Belle knew they were near their destination by the barking and baying of the hounds.

They stopped at the door of a small cabin that was well hidden with mountain laurel and pine. Belle shook the rain from her coat, and the man stepped in and held the lantern high. She could see the form of a man lying upon on a bed near the back wall. The man who brought her here stirred the dying fire and Belle went to get a glimpse of her patient.

He was struggling with each breath and Belle placed her hand on his head to check his temperature. She laid an ear to his chest and heard raspy lungs. She checked his pulse and looked at his pupils, knowing that his time was running out and not knowing if she could pull him through. She turned around to talk to the other man who stood silently by. "I believe he has lung fever, or pneumonia. I will do what I can for him, but he's been sick for sometime, I believe." She placed two pillows beneath his head to elevate him and straightened his blanket.

The man shook his head and said, "Is there anything I can do?"

"Keep the fire goin' and bring in some water. I'll stay by him through the night and see if he improves. If you could find some flat rocks that are not too large, bring them in and warm them by the fire." She bathed his face and hands in lukewarm water, then took a bottle of camphor and applied it to his chest and the soles of his feet. She removed a bundle of flannel, heated it before the fire and laid it on his chest. She put a pair of wool socks on his feet. Next she wrapped the rocks in pieces of flannel and placed them at his feet. He was resting better, but he still was in an unconscious state.

She went over to the little cook stove and boiled some water, then crushed some mullein leaves and added the water. She then placed the cups of the herb all around his bed because she believed the vapors would help his breathing.

She made herself a hot tea and sat through the night by his bed. Every time he thrashed around, she replaced his blankets and she checked to see if his fever was breaking. Finally, the fever broke and the restless man grew quiet. She changed his clothes and remade the bed. She talked to him and told him to help her by lifting his arms so that she could replace his wet clothing. He fell into a deep sleep and she dozed off in the chair. When she awakened the following morning, she realized that he was looking at her. "Well, I see you made it through the night," she said.

"Who are you and how did you find me?" he asked in a raspy voice.

"Your friend fetched me here; didn't think I'd make it once or twice."

"Not many have come here; I have been alone here for several years."

"The young man said you was pretty old, but in the daylight I can see you are not old at all! That beard and hair just make you appear so. I'd better quit talking and fix you something hot to drink."

She scurried to the stove to heat some water and pour it over some leaves to steep.

When she strained the tea, she added a teaspoon of honey and a shot of whiskey and mixed it well. The man was grateful for the drink.

She noticed a heavy door at the back of the room and asked the man where it led. "It is connected to a cave where I get my water, and I store food back there. Go on back and you can find something to fix." She took a candle and a large bowl and opened the door; it was like stepping into a cellar. She could hear the water dripping and she spotted some ledges that held canned food. A box was filled with potatoes and another with apples. She dropped a few potatoes into the bowl, found an onion and a can of peaches. She was surprised at how clever he had been, building the cabin into the cliff. He could even stable animals in here if he wanted; there was plenty of room. She stoked the fire and boiled some water while she peeled and diced the potatoes and onion.

Soon the aroma of potato soup filled the air. It had been a long time since the man had eaten. When Belle had the soup in a cup, she took some to the man and helped him sit up. While he ate, she opened the peaches and mashed them in their heavy syrup. She fixed a bowl of soup for herself and sat down to talk to the man.

"Why are you here in this Godforsaken place?" she asked.

He took his time answering, as if he was thinking what to tell her. "Granny, I was married to a beautiful woman. We lived south of here. I worked the mines and built us a home. I wanted to give her anything she wanted. One day I came home from work and found her in bed with another man; I went crazy and killed them both before I stopped. I finally came to myself and lit out of there and never looked back. I have stayed mostly to myself here, living as a hermit. The boy discovered me two years ago when he got lost hunting. We have been friends since then. He brings me some store-bought food and we visit. He tells me the news of the world. I hunt and glean my foods from the woods; you are one of a few who I have seen since I came here."

"Don't you ever want to go back and see what happened?"

"No, that life is behind me now. I don't have to watch my back all the time. I am content to stay here until my life is over—which could have been sooner—if you had not happened along."

"You have pneumonia but I think you're through the worst and will make it now. I'm going to leave you some medicine and if you will take care of yourself and rest you will be well soon. Don't get out in the cold air. Your lungs are still weak, and will be so for a while. If you need me, send the boy."

"I really don't know how to thank ye, Granny; I don't have any money to pay ye."

"Did I ask ye for money? I wouldn't be takin' care of people if it was for the money. Not many around here do have money. Just get well."

She gathered her belongings and went to tell the man good-bye. When she shook his hand, he looked up and said, "You still don't know my name."

"No, I don't, and I have never met you," she said smugly as she walked out to the young man waiting to take her home.

When they started off the mountain, Belle could see that they were on the top of a huge rock cliff, densely covered with mostly hemlock with some small bushes of mountain laurel beneath. Some looked like leatherwood and there was also plenty of beech. The trail was just as hard going down as it had been going up, but at least they were in the daylight. She could see why no one had found the man. It was slow going down. She had to turn her feet sideways and dig into the wet ground. She also grabbed at some brush to support herself.

When they were traveling toward Belle's home, the man said, "I want to thank you for coming out. I have a dollar I want to pay you for your trip."

"Just keep your dollar, young man, and if you need me again, come get me," she said as she climbed out of the car. "I'll walk from here," she said. Without another word, she slammed the door and turned down the mountain toward home.

The man looked on with a smile on his face and a shake of his head. "I like that woman," he thought, as he turned toward home.

PROGRESS COMES TO THE MOUNTAINS

Winter had once again taken its grip on the mountain, so Belle and George stayed close to home. Belle worked on her quilts, and she and George stayed near the fire, feeding it constantly with wood and coal. They had a pet groundhog that they kept in the house. They had cut a hole in the floor near the fireplace; the groundhog would go down the hole and sleep near the fireplace and came out to play with Belle and George when they sat near the fire.

Progress had finally reached the mountains and hollows with the coming of the electricity. It took a lot of time and manpower to string wire across the high mountain peaks and down into the valleys that were densely populated. Virgin timber had to be cut and the stringing of wires followed. The wires reached Belle and George and the electric was installed in the summer of 1949.

With electricity, their way of life improved greatly. They no longer had to burn the kerosene lamps; they could work later in the evening burning the electric lights. They bought a radio at the store and gave it a special place near their fireplace. They hovered around it for news, preaching and music; they never missed the Grand Ole Opry out of Tennessee or *Amos and Andy*. It became their favorite time of day.

Radar got out of hand once while they were all listening to the new radio. He came in with an ax and crushed the radio with one swing. Another time, he was mad at his father and hit him in the head with a stick of firewood. He also tried to stab his father with a butcher knife.

Belle treated Radar's spells with Virginia snake root, an herb that the Native Americans of the area had introduced to the first settlers. It was valuable because it was widely used for many illnesses. New settlers relied more upon the medical advice of the Indians. Belle brewed the root into a tea that had a calming effect on those who drank it. But sometimes Radar still got out of hand.

SPRING, WONDERFUL SPRING

When spring finally arrived in the holler, Belle welcomed it by throwing open the windows and doors and cleaning everything inside. Sparse trees of redbud burst forth with vivid bloom. They graced the cliffs of rock along the hills, while fresh white blooms spread across the branches of the dogwood trees around Belle's farm. The fragrant scents of new flowers blew across the land, and the bright yellow bloom of forsythia announced that spring had finally arrived. Belle swept and scrubbed the wooden floors, cleaned the windows with a solution of vinegar and water, and dried them with crumbled newspapers.

She was feeling renewed herself when she walked to the cellar and cleaned out the bins of potatoes and apples. She left some potatoes for seed and she took a bucket of the culls to the pigpen. She hollered, "Suey, suey," and the pigs came running to the trough. She then checked on her old horse and laid down some new hay in the stall. She curried the horse and noticed some gray in her coat. "Well, old girl, I wonder who will last the longest," she said with a laugh. She gave her a couple of sugar cubes from her pocket and patted her on the head; Old Boss kicked up her heels. When Belle got outside the horse shed, she kicked up her heels, too. Warm weather was on its way.

She walked to the smokehouse and checked the meat that was hanging inside. She cut a huge slab of ham and took it inside to cook.

Spring revivals sprang up at all the churches and Belle, Cordelia, Marilda and her sister Leslie tried to attend as many as they could. At the last service of the week, on Sunday afternoon, the congregation had dinner on the grounds.

Belle caught a couple of chickens and cut off their heads. She gutted them and scalded them in hot water and went about plucking the feathers. When they were clean and bare, she put them on to cook for a big pot of chicken and dumplings. It was always everyone's favorite and she meant to have plenty to share. Marilda would fix stack apple pies and Cordelia would bring many of her canned goods from her cellar to add. Leslie liked to make cakes; she also brought foods from her cellar. There was nothing like the renewing of the spirit and enjoying the bounty of a big meal all on the same day.

HONEY!!!

In late summer Belle and George hunted for a bee tree. Their supply of honey was running low and needed to be replenished. They followed the bees and could see a colony working in swarms. They marked the tree and watched it until it was ready to rob. They believed that the bees did not attack as bad if they first took a bath to remove the human smell. They dressed in long-sleeved clothes and tied all the openings so no bee could get in. Belle had fashioned two large hats with brims, adding a veil of netting over the face and down to the shirt opening.

They collected the items needed and took a large washtub to carry the honey home. They arrived early at the bee tree, because the bees would not swarm as much early in the day. The honey and combs were inside a large beech that had a hollow center. It was high in the tree and they had to fashion a ladder to the tree by nailing strong sticks across the trunk. They had brought along a torch and some kerosene. George climbed the tree and pushed the burning torch into the tree until he saw the bees coming out. They sat down to watch. When the swarm had left, Belle climbed the tree and began to load part of the honey into buckets. She handed the buckets off to George and he sent up the next bucket while he emptied the full one into the tub.

A few bees swarmed around, but Belle and George were safely covered. When a couple stray bees swarmed angrily around her head, Belle would use the canister smoker to drive them away. When the tub was nearly full, George told her to take some comb out and come down. Belle filled one more bucket with comb and honey and placed everything back as it was so the bees would return and make more honey for their winter stay. She knew that you never robbed the entire hive.

Belle and George carried the tub and all of their tools toward home. They were sticky, tired, and satisfied that they had brought enough out for the winter. When they got home they removed the heavy clothes and washed the honey from their hands. Belle had sanitized half-gallon jars and they packed them with comb and honey. They had to pick out a dead bee now and then, but the honey smelled so good they only thought about the taste.

When they had packed all the jars and cleaned the tub and tools, George went to the creek with a bar of soap and a towel and washed the honey away. Belle heated water and took a quick warm bath. People in the mountains used honey for most of their sweetening. Some people called it "sase" or long sweeten.

MIDWIFE DUTIES

Belle worked less now as a midwife. As time progressed, people had money for a doctor, so she was not in as much demand. But she still delivered for her family. Her daughter Glacie had twin girls that Belle delivered in 1947. Glac and Elk Keith lived near the Lilly School when the twin girls were born. Belle complained to Glacie that she did not take kindly to a woman in labor sitting up in bed and smoking. But Glac just waved her hand as if to say 'oh well.'

An older daughter of Glacie's, Chessie, was attending school the day the twins were born. Two boys from school took a bucket to the Keith house to get water for the school. When they returned Chessie said they were telling everyone about two new babies that were born that day. Chessie was so excited she could not wait to go home and see her new sisters.

Belle never turned down a plea to help deliver babies. She was notified that a woman at Red Row was expecting a baby and they would need her services. She knew which house it was and she went down to visit with the mother and see how the pregnancy was going. When she walked in and saw the woman she asked her when she was expecting the baby. The woman said she believed that it was not due for two months but some of the other women in her neighborhood thought that she should contact a midwife now, so she had sent for Belle. As Belle examined the woman who was certainly huge, she thought she might be carrying twins. The woman had not thought of that possibility and she began to worry.

Belle told her patient to get things ready; the time had to be near since her stomach was so large. Belle went home to pack her bag and the herbs she thought she would need. She made a point of returning to the home as soon as she could. She had sent word to Annie Exline that she would like for her to come and help. If this was more than one baby, she needed skilled hands.

The husband worked at the mines and the children ranged in age from one to 16. The little house was crowded and had very little privacy, but Belle made due as she always did. After three days, Belle began to think that she might have misjudged things. She considered returning home until she heard the baby was coming, but late in the night the woman awakened Belle, who was sleeping on the living room floor, and said that her water had broken. She was having contractions and, in fact, she could hardly walk for the pressure of carrying the baby. Belle prepared a bed for the woman and awakened Annie who heated water. They both washed their hands with the green disinfectant soap. Belle gave some pads she had made to Annie and asked her to put them in the oven. Belle had checked the woman and could see the head crowning.

She got her leather straps and tied them on the foot of the bed. She moved the woman down in the bed until she could place her feet on the footboard. Belle stayed with the woman constantly now and encouraged her through the labor. When the woman's strength was nearly gone, the baby slipped into the hands of Belle Neal. She cut the cord and handed her to Annie. She was turning around to check on the patient and another baby came into her hands. She again cut the cord and was handing the baby to Annie when the mother gave another hard push and still another baby came into the world. Belle was amazed at how fast the delivery had been. She was unprepared for three babies.

These were the first triplets she had delivered! She knew now that the battle for the undersized babies would be a challenge. They seemed to be about 8 weeks early and were all small babies. Belle attended the mother while Annie cared for the babies. Annie cleaned them up, wrapped them in flannel blankets and laid them side-by-side—three girls fussing and sucking at their thumbs and crying their way into the world. Belle helped the mother as she changed the bed and gave her some fresh pillows and a warm blanket. Then they handed the babies to her. They seemed to be identical. All had dark hair and Belle guessed that they each weighed about three pounds.

Belle fixed the silver nitrate and dropped it into their eyes. Belle was explaining to the mother that the three were going to need some extra care, as they were small. She began to prepare an incubator for each one. She took a drawer from the dresser and laid a feather pillow inside, and then laid the first baby on the pillow, adding a heating bag filled with warm water at the baby's feet. She found a clothesbasket and placed the next baby inside. Finally she found a cardboard box and lined it with a pillow and warm flannel. She was talking to the woman, as she worked with the babies, saying that she needed to be very careful with these premature babies—no outside visitors and very limited outings. She told the mother that they could keep the babies warm by warming bricks and covering them well and lay them in the babies' cribs. For a while the care of the three would be a 24-hour a day job.

When Belle got home she realized that in one month she had not only brought her twin grandbabies into the world but now her first triplets!

COMPANY'S COMIN'

On a Sunday in spring, Belle rose early to start dinner. She was preparing for her children that were coming to visit. She went out to the chicken pen and picked out two plump hens. She tied their feet together and took them to the chopping block near the woodpile. She quickly beheaded the clucking hens and dipped them in scalding water. By the time the dew had dried from the grass, Belle had the chickens cut up and boiling in a large pot.

Dinner would be chicken and dumplings, fresh green beans and plenty of homemade bread, cake and pies, homemade jelly and hot coffee. Belle's mouth watered as she smelled the chicken cooking. She had rushed through the morning, but now, with everything ready, she took a pan of warm water in one of the back rooms to sponge off and change clothes. She put on a clean dress and an apron made from feed sacks. She donned her high top sneakers and combed her gray hair and twisted it into a bun at the nape of her neck. She looked in the little mirror on top of the chest of drawers and smoothed back stray hair.

As Belle was leaving the room, she wished she had not cut so much of her hair recently, but at the time she thought that it was thinning and the ends were ragged. She had not been able to part with her hair so she wrapped it in paper and placed it in the trunk where she kept her treasures.

In the top tray there was a picture of Leo, from when he had come home on leave from the service before he was killed. Sometimes she would take the picture out and look at it and still could not believe he was gone. The pictures of her great nieces and nephews also were in the tray on top. On the bottom were several quilts she had made and had not used. She thought she would save them for someone who was getting married. She liked to be prepared for something like that. She lifted a silk banner near the bottom of the trunk; it smelled of cedar and she ran her work-worn hands over it. It had been sent to her from some foreign land after Leo had returned to active duty. It was packed with a telegram edged in black that two service men had brought, telling of his death. She could get all teary-eyed but what was the use? It would not change anything. "Today and maybe tomorrow I can change, but not much beyond that," she said as she struggled to get up off of the floor and loosen her arthritic joints.

She seemed to return to the present as she headed toward the kitchen and she could hear the kids arriving. They came down the rough road, bouncing along, with the children hanging out the windows, waving and calling. George and Belle stood on the porch and waved back, waiting there with a smile on their faces. When Elk got the car stopped and the kids out, George and Belle went to pick up the twins who were nearing their second birthday.

Glacie said, "Mom and Dad, stand over there by the fence and let me get a picture of you with the twins. Then I want a picture of the girls, Chessie, Bonnie Barb and Elore and the boys Maxell, Darnell and Robert." The girls wanted their picture taken with their grandparents and then the boys had to have one too! Radar came out of the house and Glacie snapped a picture of him standing in front of their car. She worked quickly because Radar did not like having his picture taken and she didn't want him to be in a foul mood with them. Marv and Lou also came down with their children to spend the day.

"Its time to go in and wash up for dinner, kids," said Belle as she shooed them in the house. Elk, George, and Marv stayed on the porch talking while Belle and the women dished up the food and sat the kids down.

Everyone made quick haste of the food. The kids wanted to hurry so they could go outside and explore the farm. Belle and the women finally got to eat while they held the twin girls and the other babies. Belle opened the doors and windows, hoping for a breeze as they cleaned up the kitchen. After all was tidy again they went outside to sit and let the babies play on the porch. It was a beautiful summer day and Belle felt content; just spending the day with family meant so much.

"Glac, you know the fair is coming to town in about two weeks, don't ye?" asked Belle.

"Me and George is plannin' to go if we can get a ride up and back. I want to look at the canned vegetables, jellies, quilts and livestock. Shoot, me and George might even get our picture taken," laughed Belle.

"Ma, I can have Elk to come and get you, but he will have to make two trips back and up," said Glac.

"We'll be ready if ye tell us when. We might see someone there who will bring us back. Just about everyone in the county goes to the fair."

As the sun was setting and the land was cooling down, the adults started to round up their children. The kids protested that they had not had enough time to play; some were even crying. When the children were finally all on their way, Belle and George waved goodbye to them from the porch steps.

They could hear the Elk's old car spurting and protesting all the way to the top, and the voices of the families walking echoed against the hills in the holler and then the silence seemed to set in and engulf them.

George, Belle, and Radar sat on the porch not saying anything, watching the sun sink and enjoying the evening coolness. Finally, the hush of quiet was broken when a whippoorwill's comforting call rang out across the stillness. When the sun finally sank behind the hill, the darkness clothed them in great peace. The lightning bugs fluttered across the yard, and in the distance they heard the howl of Marv's coon dogs. Belle and George sat comfortably in silence savoring the day.

COUNTY FAIR

George and Belle were as excited as kids when they were planning their trip to the county fair. Belle took her bath and laid out her clean clothes. Then she went to find George some clothes to wear. She found him a pair of pinstripe navy pants and a white shirt. She added his suspenders and clean underwear. They ate a quick lunch and got themselves ready to go. They were on the porch waiting by early afternoon. Their son-in-law, Elk, came for them after he had taken his own family to the fair. Belle heard Elk's car before she saw it. "Here comes Elk, George. Better go and get your jacket and mine, too. They are on the bed. Do you have any money on ye?"

"I got enough to get in the gate; you got any extra if I need it, Belle?"

"Yell, I got some for a bit of food. Just tell me when you need some more."

They were as excited as two kids as they walked across the foot log and were waiting when Elk stopped.

Belle got in the front and George took the back seat. "Elk, I don't have to tell you to go slow. I'm not real fond of these new inventions; cain't say I'll ever get used to ridin' anything faster than a horse."

Elk drove at a slow crawl up the mountain and just smiled at Belle.

When they arrived at the fair they had to stand in line to pay. Glac and the kids had been waiting just inside and the kids came running to their grandparents. Belle took one of the babies and held the hand of another and, with Glac, headed toward the fair items on display. George went to see the livestock and walked around to see the booths that took your money.

Belle looked at the quilts and canned goods and said to Glac, as she picked up a quilt with a blue ribbon, "I believe I will enter some of my things next year. I know I can quilt better than this!" Some people standing around heard her but only laughed to themselves. If they knew Belle they knew not to comment on anything she said. When they had seen all of the exhibits, they walked around the fair and stopped to watch a man shooting a dart gun at balloons. He shot enough to let his girlfriend pick out a big stuffed animal. Belle knew that she could probably hit enough for a prize, but she didn't want to waste the money. They moved on and let the children pick up ducks for a nickel. They all got a little gift and were happy. They ran into George and Elk and they all decided to stop at a food booth and get some food. Bingo was being played, but Belle didn't believe in gambling, which she thought was the devil's own work!

They walked around some more and stopped to talk to people along the way. There was a big ferris wheel turning over and over. Belle looked up and thought if that thing would come off it would go right to the river. She had never been as high as that wheel and she planned to keep both feet on the ground, thank ye! She walked around the fairground and noticed one booth had a large line of people. She tiptoed to see what the attraction was. The large sign on the booth read: "Have your picture taken with the Wild Man." She smiled and walked on. That was her cousin Orval Brown, impressing the people, but she could have her picture taken with him anytime!

They ran into many people from their area and asked if someone could take them home. One of their nephews said he would be glad to drop them off at their road.

"Well, just come and find us when you get ready to go. Me and George have seen all we need to." They were getting tired and went to find a seat on some benches near the front. Belle noticed a booth where they were taking pictures and walked over to see how much it cost. The cost was a quarter. "George, come over here and we'll get our picture made," called Belle.

"No, you go on. I'm too tired," said George. She did get her picture taken wearing a holster with two guns and a cowboy hat!

THE FAMILY VISITS

One day Dilly's daughters from Beckley, Jane and Grace, came to visit Dilly. They knew that her health was not the best and wanted to visit with her while they could. Dilly slept in the middle room of the house in an iron bed with newspapers pasted on the wall. Aunt Belle also came to see her nieces. Cordelia's daughters, Marilda, Leslie, Jane and Grace, were all gathered in Dilly's room talking, as women will, about their bodies. Belle said her legs were white, having never being exposed to the sun.

Someone else mentioned the breast and Belle said hers were still firm and she pulled down the front of her dress and exposed her breast. Most everyone knew how Aunt Belle was and just passed it off with a laugh. But those who had not been acquainted with Belle thought it was terrible. The kids who had grown up with Aunt Belle were miffed at the others who talked badly about her. The children who knew Belle decided to fight the others for criticizing her. Belle was always supporting her great nieces and nephews and the children returned the favor for Belle.

When the city children came out of the house, the kids of the area threw rocks at them until they ran away into the woods and hid. Ann's dad, Bib, saw the kids throwing the rocks and fighting. He called Ann to come to the porch; he was going to whip Ann for her part in the fight. Aunt Belle was on the front porch with Bib and she heard him tell Ann she was being disciplined for her part in the fight. Belle told him not to whip Ann because she knew how the city children were acting and that the kids here were protecting Belle. Belle was miffed and with a smug look on her face, she shook her head and said, "I will get them little hussies!" Belle sat down to think what she could do to teach the city kids a lesson in respect. Those children did not know what they were in for!

HOMECOMING DAY

By late September the year's bounty was ready for harvest. It was gathered at the time the church planned a homecoming with dinner outside on the grounds. Marlida would make stack apple pies and Leslie would fry up a pan of chicken. Belle usually fixed a chocolate cake and lemon pies, but she wanted to make something different this year. She had to think on it and make sure she had supplies on hand.

She believed she had a smoked ham in the smokehouse. "Now, that would go good," she thought, "if I could fix a little brown sugar drizzle and bake it up real tender. Why, yeah! That is what I'll fix and maybe an apple cake." She went out to the smokehouse and made sure that the ham was indeed there. It was and she felt content knowing it was there. She never liked to wait 'til the last minute to get things done.

Saturday before the homecoming dawned bright, with just a hint of fall in the air. The leaves were starting to turn bright reds, gold, orange and yellow. Doing outside chores this time of year was so relaxing; it was Belle's favorite time of year. She was shucking the last of the corn and laying them in a bushel basket. She cleaned them of silks and then laid the shucks and stocks in a pile to take to the barn. The corn had done really well this year and she and Radar had made two churns of pickled corn. Then she had canned up 25 half-gallons. These nubs that were the last harvest would be cooked, then buttered and salted and taken to the church tomorrow.

Belle could see Radar across the road working in the garden. He was pulling the last of the corn stocks and tying them into fodder. When the first frost touched the pumpkins they would roll them inside the fodder. They had dug over 100 lbs of potatoes and they were safely in the cellar, along with the canned vegetables and churns of corn and kraut. It looked like Radar was doing a good job so she finished up the corn and took the scraps to her hogs. They had finally been penned up a few weeks ago. Until then, they had roamed the forest as free spirits, living off the mast of the fall. Belle thought it best if they fed them these last few weeks before the butchering.

She looked in on Old Boss, who had retired from the job of carrying Belle through the hills. They both needed a long rest. She threw some corncobs to the horse and some fodder to the cow. She had a young calf that had been born in spring. She was thinking that she would give it to her granddaughter, Chessie. "As long as someone had a cow they would never be without milk," she thought.

Belle arose early on homecoming day. She had prepared the ham the night before and now she warmed it in the oven. She had baked a delicious apple cake that was moist and crunchy with the small pieces of walnut she had added. This morning she was fixing a glaze that she would pour over the cake which would soak in. She put a big kettle of water on the stove and let it come to a boil. Then she placed the corn on the cob inside and let it boil for ten minutes. Next, she looked for a wooden crate that she kept to pack her food in. She finally found it turned upside down on the back stoop. She cleaned it up and poured scalding water over it and let it set in the sun to dry. She returned to the stove and removed the ham, then wrapped it in newspapers. She drained the corn and laid it back in the hot pot and covered it with a clean dishtowel. She drizzled the cake after she punched holes in the top with a fork. She stuck toothpicks into the top and wrapped the cake in newspaper and then clean towels.

Belle went to get herself ready for church. She had everything ready when Homer and Forest came down the mountain to take her to the church. They had purchased an old Dodge truck that they used when they cut posts to haul them to the mill to sell. The truck wasn't much; it was rusted and old but it was all they could afford. The driver's door was wired shut so they had to crawl out the passenger side.

"Hello, Aunt Belle," said Homer, "Mony sent me and Forest to get you to the church."

Forest was already carrying her food to the truck, "I'll ride in the back, Aunt Belle. Do you need some help gettin' in?"

"No, no. I can make it," she said as she pulled a little dark blue hat down on her head and crawled up in the seat.

"I don't know what you fixed to eat, but it sure smells good," said Homer as he sniffed the air. "I fixed plenty of extra. You know how it is on homecoming day. We have so many that don't bring food and the rest of us have to prepare for that." Homer shook his head that he understood. They finally got turned around and were climbing up the steep hill slowly.

Forest was holding on in the back. He was sitting on the spare tire and holding on to the sides of the truck, trying to keep the food from bouncing.

When they reached their home at the bottom of the mountain, they stopped and went to get Marilda and Cordelia's food. Homer drove with Belle and Cordelia up front. Marilda and Forest and all the little kids rode in the back. When Homer looked in his rear view mirror, he could see heads sticking out everywhere.

They arrived at church as everyone was going in. Homer and Forest stayed outside and put the lunch baskets in the shade of a large sycamore tree. People came in from every direction—walking, some riding in cars, and others coming in wagons. After the morning service, the women began to spread the food on large tables made for the homecoming.

Kids played on the hill behind the school, riding down to the bottom on cardboard; others cut a grapevine and took turns swinging out over the creek. The young men and women sat around getting to know each other and the older people moved about the crowd talking to first one, then another. Everyone went inside the schoolhouse to have a final service of the day. They raised the rafters as they sang the old gospel songs: *When They Ring Those Golden Bells*, *Precious Memories* and *The Old Gospel Ship*; people felt very close to God when they attended services and when they sang those special songs.

When the services ended, people packed their picnic baskets away and headed for home. Their bodies and their souls had been fed.

TRAVELING GRANNY

On a hot summer day, Belle was walking out Beechy Ridge on her way to a home where a woman was expecting a baby. Belle had promised to be there for the birth. She climbed a steep part of the rutted road and she was hot and tired. She could see that she was near the Davis house and thought she would stop for a drink of water. She hollered at the road and a woman and several children came out on the porch. "I would like a cold drink of water, Ms. Davis."

The woman was wiping her hands on her apron. "Sure, sure, come on in," she said, "Son, get us some cool water," she said to a teenager. "Where are you headed, Belle?"

"I promised Sadie Markle that I would be there to deliver her next born baby. I see that you have had a lot of cherries this year; looks like the trees were loaded down," Belle said as she pointed to the trees in the yard.

"Yes, we have had a good crop and we have canned for several weeks now. They are almost gone." The boy brought them both a glass of water and they sat in silence for a while.

"Well, I guess I'll mosey on to the Markle's. I want to get there before dark," said Belle.

"Be sure and stop by on your way home and tell us about the baby," said Ms. Davis as she waved Belle goodbye.

"I will, and thanks for the water," said Belle as she resumed her walk out the ridge. As Belle walked around the ridge she could see people walking toward her and when they met in the road, they stopped to talk. The old woman was Lenore Schoonover. She was dressed in a long black dress and a sunbonnet. She walked with a cane and was stooped and bent. The young woman was her granddaughter Betty and they were headed for Glen, where their relatives lived.

Belle said, "I hope you don't plan to get there in one day Ms. Schoonover."

"No, we walk awhile and stop and visit people along the way. Sometimes it takes me about three days to get there."

"Well, you all be careful now," said Belle and they headed in opposite directions. "That woman sure is a determined woman!" thought Belle.

When Belle arrived at the Markle's she could hear music coming through the open windows. She stepped upon the porch and could see the children dancing and laughing around a Victrola. Sadie saw Belle on the porch and she rushed to the door and opened it wide. Sadie looked like she was carrying twins and she had a time just walking around. The children became aware of a visitor and became very quiet.

"Don't stop on my account," said Belle, "Go ahead and sing." She was hoping that they would put some more music on. It was the first Victrola she had ever seen and she hoped the children would play it again.

Sadie told Belle to sit down and rest and one of the kids brought her some water.

"How you feelin', Sadie? It looks like it won't be long."

Sadie rubbed her stomach and said, "Sure hope so. It's hard to carry around this extra weight."

Belle said, "I knew if I didn't come, you would be all alone with the children with Jim working away."

"I'm sure glad you are here, Belle. I was just about to put the supper on. Come into the kitchen and talk to me there."

They had a pot of fresh green beans, new potatoes, hot cornbread and some crisp fried bacon. When supper was over, Belle helped the girls clean up the kitchen and then she went to make herself a bed in the upstairs room that the girls shared. They went out onto the porch and enjoyed the quietness of a summer's eve while the lightning bugs floated around and the children ran to catch them. The beautiful sunset left red rays across the sky and the sounds of the birds settling in for the night made for a relaxing evening.

When Belle rose the following morning she started the coffee and breakfast. She checked on her patient and was pleased to find Sadie sleeping; she would need her rest. The oldest girl and boy came down the stairs and Belle told them that they were going to help her clean the house and do the laundry. They started with the living room, removing the rag rugs. The girl took them outside to beat them clean.

The boy cleaned the fireplaces and Belle swept down the walls and the floor. Then they scrubbed the wooden floors with hot bleach water. By the time the living room was cleaned and dusted, the smaller children came for breakfast. While the oldest daughter fixed their breakfast, Belle went to gather the bed sheets and clothing. Sadie's oldest son helped her build a fire under the big kettle and Belle scrubbed and cleaned until the laundry was done. She sat down on the back steps and fanned herself. In a while, Jane, the oldest girl, brought her a wet towel and some cold water.

Belle had been going in at intervals to check on Sadie. She was awake when Belle looked in and asked her how she was feeling. Sadie said she didn't think she should get up and walk around because the baby felt different today. Belle assumed that the baby had moved into the birth canal. "Just rest, Sadie, and we'll take care of the children. I'll have Jane bring you a light breakfast."

All through the day Belle looked in on her patient and knew that she would probably spend the night sitting by Sadie's side. After a busy day of work and caring for the children, Belle felt stiff and old, but she pulled up a rocker and dozed off and on through the night. When morning came she got things ready for the newborn. She heard the children playing outside and was glad that they were well occupied. She heard Jim as he came inside and Belle went to see him.

"Jim, you're a day early, ain't ye?"

"Yell, I thought I'd come home from the timber job and check on the family."

"Glad you made it. You can watch the children while I watch Sadie. I expect you'll need to make yourself a bed on the couch tonight."

"Could I go in and see Sadie and let her know I'm home?"

"Yell, go ahead while I boil some water and lay out some supplies."

Belle opened her doctor's bag and found the corn silk. She sterilized her scissors and needles with boiling water. She soaked her thread in alcohol and then sweet oil; she laid some heavy pads in the oven to sterilize them. She removed a jar of lard she kept to use for a lubricant. She poured herself a pan of hot water and scrubbed her hands with the green soap she carried. She took everything to Sadie's room and to see how her patient was doing. Sadie was having some hard pains and she was nearly exhausted.

Belle rubbed Sadie's lips with some cool water and wiped her face with a damp cloth. After a pain had ended, Belle said she needed to do an examination. Belle could tell the time was nearing for the birth. She could see the baby's head and she watched through two more pains, but still the head did not move down. Belle told Sadie that she was going to pull the baby out on her next pain. She thought that it was big and its shoulders were keeping it from moving. Sadie was so relieved that she readily agreed.

Belle said, "Sadie, when I tell you to push, give it all you've got. Okay, I am going to slide my hands on the shoulders and you help me. Now let's bring him out." He came into the world screaming with lustful cries; he had been freed from his warm place. Belle snipped the cord after tying it off and laid him on his mother's breast.

Belle worked swiftly to knead the afterbirth and she could see that Sadie would need some stitches. She got her needle and thread and stitched Sadie up. Then she placed a poultice of corn silk over the stitches. She placed the warm pads between her legs and a thick layer of sheets beneath her and covered her with a warm blanket. She then took the baby and dropped the nitrate into the eyes and wrapped him in a blanket. "I believe this one is near big as his daddy," she laughed and said, as she handed the baby to the mother, "What are you going to name him?"

"I was thinking George after my father."

"That's good. You know, my man is named George."

Belle took the afterbirth to the man and told him to bury it and then he could come in and see the baby. After the man came back, they called the children to come meet their new brother. Then Belle ran them all out and proceeded to take care of the child and mother. "I tell you, Sadie, I thought I was delivering Jim. This is such a big boy! He is going to have a hefty start in life. I think he weighs about 10 pounds."

Belle piddled around the bedroom, putting everything in order. While the woman and child slept, Belle went to fix herself something to eat. She talked with Jim, who was sitting in the living room.

"I want to thank you for coming and taking care of my family, Ms. Neal. I knew that I could not make it home and I hated to leave the children here alone while their mother was in labor. I just don't know how to thank you."

"I always think that this is my job. I try to get to the homes when I can to help the most. I will be leaving in the morning, though. I hope you will be here for a few days to help the children."

The following morning Belle rose early, fixed some breakfast, and then looked in on her patients. She registered the date and sex of the child and names of the mother and father. She was now required by law to record and submit the baby's identity to the county clerk's office.

Belle gathered up her belongings and said a hurried goodbye to the children. Sadie told Belle that a young couple had moved into a large two-story house in Beechy, near the school. She said she had only met the people once and the young girl was expecting a baby. She and Sadie both had been concerned that she could not get out to find a doctor or midwife. Sadie had promised to let Belle know about the woman. Belle assured Sadie that the husband could come and get her when the time was near.

She walked along, thinking over the past few days. When she finally got to the Davis home, she remembered she was supposed to stop by and tell them of the baby. She walked up on the porch and hollered inside. The woman and children came and asked about the baby. They brought her some fresh water and she sat down for a few minutes. When she had rested, she started on her way home. Walking out the ridge road, she looked back and saw the Davis' watching her go. When she reached the place in the road they called the Rocky Low Gap, she heard a car sputtering and rattling along. She moved over to the edge of the road and the car stopped. It was the Kings from over on the other ridge. They wanted to give her a ride home. The car was loaded down with children sticking their heads out the windows. Belle handed her bag inside and stepped up on the running board. They talked to her all the way.

She was thinking how good country people could be. They had saved her a long walk. She arrived home and decided to take a sponge bath and lay down for a while. When she awakened, Radar was preparing supper. Belle didn't say much; she was just too tired to talk. They passed a nice evening just resting.

A CALL FOR THE DOCTOR

Belle had just changed into her nightclothes one summer evening and was about to turn out the light when she heard a car bouncing down her road. She stepped out onto the porch and waited to see if it was she they needed. A young man she could not identify stretched his long frame out of the old truck and headed toward her house. When he reached the foot log, Belle stepped out onto the steps and said, "What can I do for you, young feller?"

He was surprised to see her standing right in front of him and he drew back a little.

"Are you a granny woman?" he asked.

"Some call me that; I go by the name of Belle Neal."

"Well, you are the one I am looking for then. My mother is very sick and I was told to ask if you would see her."

"Do you live a far piece from here? I don't believe I've seen you in these parts," Belle questioned him.

"No, I just moved to Blue Knob. I have been trying to farm the land. My mother has been sick for sometime now and I don't know what to do for her. I had her to the doctor in Clay, but nothing has helped her. She just seems to be slipping away. She has a lot of coughing and she is very weak—coughing up blood at times."

"You come in and wait on the porch and I'll change clothes and get my doctor's bag. It won't take me long."

Belle hunted up some extra clothes and made sure the doctor's bag was packed. When she had everything ready, she wrote a short note to George and said not to look for her to return for a couple of days. She closed the door and turned the lights off. She and the man walked back to his truck in silence. He carried the bag and put it in the back while Belle climbed in front with him. She questioned him about the ailment as they drove along.

He came from up in the northern part of West Virginia. His father had died last year and he moved his mother in with him. He thought that they could work a little farm and he would provide for his mother. They had been here for nearly a month, and his mother just took to her bed with the illness and he was beginning to worry.

As they wound around the country roads that climbed a hill, they came upon a little farm. He stopped, helped her get out and took Belle in to introduce her to his mother. The house was dark except for low-burning kerosene light. He turned on more light and Belle saw the woman lying on a bed near the fireplace. She could hear her troubled breathing before she got near her. She fashioned a sock for a mask before she walked over to the bed. Belle introduced herself and told her why she had come.

The woman didn't say much and Belle didn't know if she was alert. Belle felt her skin, which was clammy, and she dropped her head to her chest and listened to her breathing. She got a pan of warm water and helped her sponge off. The woman's clothes were damp so Belle helped her change clothes. She could see that the woman was very thin and her color was gray.

After Belle changed the bed, she covered the woman with a blanket, placed two pillows behind her head, and placed her in a reclining position. She went over to the kitchen area and heated some water. While she waited for the water to boil, she removed herbs from her bag and ground them with her hands. She fixed some crushed mullein and hot water and placed a small amount in several jar lids and placed them around the sick bed. It gave off a vaporizing odor that helped breathing. She fixed a toddy with some sulfur, a teaspoon of whiskey and a dab of cane syrup. She mixed it with hot water and stirred to blend; when it had cooled, she gave it to the patient with a teaspoon. When the toddy was gone, the woman slipped back off to sleep and Belle began to rummage through the food items. She found enough vegetables to make a pot of soup. As it simmered on the stove she realized she was very hungry.

The young man came in the door after he had taken care of his farm animals. They spoke in quiet tones, so as not to wake his mother.

"Ms. Neal, I forgot to tell you my mother's name. It's June. Do you have an idea of what is wrong with her?"

"I cain't rightly say, but I am afeared that it is lung fever or TB; she is spitting up some blood. If that is the case, there is not a lot I can do for her. I'll stay the night and see what I can come up with in the morning. You will have to get someone to attend her through the day while you work and few are willing to place their selves in this situation. You know that it is an airborne disease and very contagious. It is really a matter of time as to the outcome of this illness. It might be a long time, with her just wasting away."

The following morning the young man made a trip around the ridge and found a woman who would come during the day while he worked. She had buried a sister whom she had nursed with TB so she knew the danger but she needed the money and so a deal was struck. Belle warned her to wear a mask and wash her hands constantly.

"Well, that is about all I can do except leave her some herbs that could be used to help her some. I better get back home before my man comes looking for me."

She went over and held the woman's hand and told her she was leaving but there was someone who would be staying with her. The woman thanked her even though it took all of the energy that she had. Belle gave her a pat and walked away, knowing that there was not much anyone could do for this illness.

A BAPTIZING AT THE SCHOOL

School had started in late September and the children were playing on the grounds. They were having church, as children will do. A Neal boy of about 12 was the preacher and Ann Osborne was the song leader. After a hell, fire and brimstone service that brought all the children to repentance, the group decided to have a baptizing. They went down to the creek and began damming up a good place. They were really getting serious and the children were standing in line to be baptized.

Someone had informed Ms. Reed, the teacher, about the event of the day. Ms. Reed soon broke up the service and made all of the children involved go in and sit in their seats. Leonard Neal, who was a fast runner, saw Belle Neal at the store near the school and ran to tell her what was happening. Belle did not like that one bit. She was rallied now and set out for the schoolhouse as fast as she could go. The farther she walked, the madder she got and when she arrived at the school, she stuck her finger up under the teacher's nose and said, "If they are being punished for playing church, the teacher is the one needin' help!"

The teacher realized that when someone did an injustice to the children, they could look to Belle Neal to come to their aid. Belle spoke her piece and went to find herself a seat. Much to the discomfort of Ms. Reed, Belle remained in the classroom until it was closed for the day. Belle was not always liked by people due to her blunt ways, but when someone mistreated children, they could be certain that she would intervene.

VISITIN' AN OLD FRIEND

Belle got to thinkin' about an old woman who lived alone on a mountaintop near Bickmore. She decided to go pay the old gal a visit before the weather got bad. She gathered some potatoes and a few jars of home canned food. She took along her doctor's bag and a change of clothes. She saddled up Old Boss and they traveled south on Route 16 until she came to a road up the mountain. She rode slowly to spare Old Boss and to watch for briars that extended out along the trail. It was a path that few traveled. Belle continued a steady climb as she rode around the mountain, taking many switchbacks along the way. She stopped about halfway up and let 'Boss' take a rest. She walked out on the edge of the mountain path and looked down on Route 16.

She hadn't traveled far but it seemed to be another world up here on the mountain. It certainly was peaceful and quiet; about the only foreign sounds were the explosions from the mines when they blasted for coal. Belle wiped her face with the edge of her apron and decided to move on. She walked awhile and let Boss carry the rest. They were walking along the rutted and rocky road when they came to an area surrounded by dense woodland. Belle stopped and looked down on a piece of land that looked like a modern day football field. She stood looking at what appeared to be a deep bowl. She wondered if some illegal act such as moonshining could be hidden there.

It was secluded on an isolated mountain where travel was at a minimum, unlikely to be discovered by the law. But if some illegal act was taking place, she could no doubt name the owners. When she turned a sharp curve near the top of the mountain, she could see a little log cabin setting beneath the grove of huge oak trees. The cabin had been here so long that it seemed a natural part of the forest. The porch of the cabin was nearly covered by thick growing vines, the tin roof was rusted and foliage of mountain laurel almost masked the cabin from view.

Belle got within a 100 feet of the cabin and she stopped and yelled "hello". Grace's old blue-tick hound appeared from under the porch, growling and showing his hackles. She knew better than to come upon the cabin without announcing herself. The old woman who lived here would shoot first and ask questions later.

In a short time Belle could see movement on the porch and then the old woman came down the steps carrying her shotgun. When she recognized Belle, she waved her on in, telling Old Blue to hush. When Belle got near the porch she looked over at Granny Grace. She hadn't changed since their last visit—still wearing her old black sunbonnet and her apron, toting her old gun by her side.

"Howdy, Belle! I sure wasn't expectin' you. How ye' been?"

"I'm doing alright Grace. I swear I don't believe you age like the rest of us. I had a dream about you the other night and I said to myself, "I need to visit Grace and see how she goes.""

"Come in, come in and I'll fix us some cold tea."

Belle tied the horse to a post, removed all the items, and placed them on the porch. Things seem about the same here, she thought as she sat down in a rocker on the front porch to rest. She believed that Grace must have been baking a cake; the aroma coming from inside the cabin made her mouth water. Soon Grace came out with the tea and they sat down and talked for a while. Belle told Grace how things were in the community and Grace just seemed to let it soak in. She had very few visitors and never went off the mountain herself.

"Grace, how long have you lived on this mountain?" Belle asked.

"I been here since 1925. Me and my man came in here to farm. We loved it here and thought we wouldn't need anything else, as long as we had each other. The first years were good. We planted an orchard here on top of the mountain. We raised our own food and he hunted for game. We were so satisfied that we didn't need to go off the mountain; most every thing we needed was here. Things went real good for the first few years and then Ralph was cutting down a tree and it fell on him and killed him instantly. I have been here by myself ever since. I buried him up there on that knoll," she gestured toward the hill.

"I used to go there every day, but now I do well to get around in the house. This was not what I had planned for old age, but I don't have anywhere else to go. I can depend on the orchard, though, I lease it out and the people come in and take care of it, then sell the fruits," Grace said as she looked out over the mountain and rocked in her chair. The sadness of remembering was hard for her, but she didn't let it last for long.

"So what brings you here, Belle?"

"Oh I don't know, just thinking about you and wantin' to come before cold weather. I just needed to know you were alright."

"I've been alright here for a long time. One of the boys from the store comes in about every two weeks and brings me groceries. I get a load of coal and wood every fall and I make out all right. But I sure do like to see somebody now and then; are you goin' stay the night?"

"Yell, I thought I might. I've not been so busy deliverin' babies right now and I needed a break anyway."

"I was getting ready to fix myself some supper. Let's go in and I'll put some bread in the oven and we can talk while it bakes. I just took a pound cake out of the oven."

Belle remembered that she had brought some canned food and went to get them from her sack on the porch. She had brought some hot peppers and onions that she and Cordelia always made in the fall. They were delicious alone, but best when eaten with beans or soups. She had brought her some turnips and cans of blackberries to make a pie or jelly. Grace was happy to get the food and she wanted Belle to take a load of apples home with her. When supper was over and everything was in its place, they returned to the porch. Grace brought out her dulcimer and began to strum the old instrument. She began the story of Barbree Allen and Belle joined in on the verses she knew. They sang a few old gospel songs and before the sun went down, Belle went out to feed and water Boss.

They went inside and lit a lantern and Grace brought out the quilts she had made last winter. Belle loved to look at the handiwork and the scheme of colors that Grace had used in the quilts. She also told her about quilts she had made and promised to bring her some patterns. They talked late into the night and finally Belle made herself a bed on the sofa. "It sure is peaceful here," Belle thought, and that was the last thing she thought until she smelled coffee the next morning.

They had a wonderful breakfast. Grace made hot biscuits and creamed tomatoes and bacon. It was so good to be here and they both enjoyed the visit.

Grace was nearing her 90th birthday and she did not get around as well as she used to. Belle asked her to get someone to come and live with her that could help her. Grace promised to think about it and Belle felt better for mentioning the idea.

They climbed up the knoll to Ralph's gravesite; Belle helped Grace along slowly. They stayed and visited for a while. Belle pulled all the high weeds from around the headstone and they placed a few wildflowers on the grave. Then they gathered a bushel of apples and Belle tied them in a burlap sack.

"I don't know what is goin' on here Belle, but I believe some people are up to no good," she pointed toward the mountain in the distance. "I have been seeing some lights over on the west side at night. I can't hear anything but the lights are there, moving around every night."

"Might be some fellars makin' moonshine; it would be a good spot away from the local road and all. I'm goin' to be worried about you. I hope they won't cause you any harm," said Belle.

"I'm not too worried; I have been on this place for a long time and no harm has come to me yet. I'm careful though. I keep this loaded shotgun with me all the time. More than likely, it is a man with a big family and needing some hard cash. If I don't bother them, maybe they won't bother me."

"Well, nonetheless, I am goin' ask someone to come and check it out," said Belle.

"I sure have enjoyed your visit, Belle. I hope that you will come back and stay a while again," Grace said.

"I will and I'll be worried until I know better. I think you ought to leave this mountain or get someone up here. I won't be satisfied until you do. I know you won't go, so we have to hope for the best. I'll see you soon," said Belle as she rode away.

Belle thought about what Grace had told her as she rode home. She kept her eyes open as she traveled the road and she could see some beaten brush just off the road. She got down off the horse and examined the trees. Whoever used this made sure to block the path with brush and fresh cut limbs. She walked around the path and slipped silently around the bowl on the mountain. She saw a huge rock that had an overhang with a dry shelter beneath. Not wanting to be seen, she watched from the dense woodland. She never did see anyone, but she was certain that it was a moonshine still. She saw some 5-gallon crock jars lined up under the rock and some glass jars on a shelf near the fire. She could smell the pungent odor of sour mash and a faint smell of burnt wood. Not wanting to get caught, she slipped back through the woods and headed on home. She did plan to notify someone to check the still. She didn't want Granny Grace to be in danger.

On a brisk February morning while the sun was shining brightly, Belle stepped out on her porch to see how warm it was outside. She was hoping for a warm day to work outside, but decided it was a little too brisk. She noticed a group of robins on the ground and knew that spring could not be far behind.

She reached for her doorknob to go back in, but suddenly felt a presence around her that made her hair stand on end. She turned to see what was there but did not see anyone; she went through the door and the mantel clock struck out the hour of ten. Next a bird hit one of the panes in the window. It rattled Belle and she was not an easy person to upset; she thought that something had happened and she was a part of it! Two days later the boy from the grocery store who delivered for Grace came by. He told her that he went to deliver groceries and he stopped and hollered before going on in to Grace's house. He knew that something was wrong when Old Blue just lay on the porch and didn't move, so he went in to the house.

Grace was propped up in bed with her Bible in her hand; she was dead. The boy said he had rushed to get someone to help him and they went in and laid her down. They were waiting for someone to prepare her for burial. Belle knew that she must go, so she thanked the boy and went to get her things together. It was a sad ride she took back to Grace's house, knowing that she would no longer be there. When she arrived some men were making a coffin and one woman waited on the porch. Belle went in and spoke to the woman and she said she would help her get ready for the burial.

Belle went in the house and removed the sheet that covered Grace. She looked so peaceful that Belle could not be sad. She believed that Grace was already with her husband and loved ones who had gone before her. She and the woman washed and dressed Grace in a dress that hung on a hook. It looked to be her best dress. They combed her hair into a bun and put a scarf around her neck. Belle laid her Bible in her hands and her sunbonnet by her side.

They waited for the men to finish the coffin. When they brought it to the porch, Belle looked at Grace one more time. The men placed her in it and then nailed the coffin shut. Someone in the neighborhood had already dug the grave. The men carried her casket to the site, lowered it in the grave, and someone said a prayer as all bowed their heads.

When the service was over, Belle headed back down the hill to the house to tidy things up before she left. There wasn't much to do, though, since Grace had been a neat person. Belle did remove the sheets from the bed and spread the quilts over it. She straightened the kitchen and threw out the churn of milk that was on the table. She cleaned the ashes from the fireplace and swept the floor. She went to a chest of drawers and tidied up the contents. Then she noticed a trunk beside the chest and she opened it to see what was inside. There were several new quilts on top, a photo album with pictures of Grace and Ralph when they married, and a few outfits of old clothes that must have been worn when they married. She found a certificate with Ralph's name stating that he had been in the 7th WV Regiment during the Civil War.

On the bottom of the chest was a small box and it had Belle's name on top. When she opened it there was a letter with Grace's handwriting. Belle was perplexed and took the letter out and held it near the window so she could read it.

Belle, I know that when I die you will be the one to take care of me and my belongings, so I am writing this letter hoping you will find it and carry out my wishes. In this box is our certificate of marriage and a little money I have saved through the years. We have no living relatives and you have been like a sister to me, so I am leaving you the money inside the box. The farm will go to the people who care for the orchard and I have nothing else worth keeping. So, to you, my dear friend, I give all I have and thank you for your friendship through the years.

Your Friend, Grace.

When Belle finished the letter, there were tears running down her cheeks. She put the letter in the box and went to the door. She looked around at the house and then closed the door and walked to her horse. All the others had long gone and the place was too quiet. Belle headed for home but before she was out of sight of the cabin, she turned back for one last look. She swore that she saw Grace standing on the porch with her shotgun and waving, with a smile on her face. Belle rode home in silence and realized that she had lost one of her dearest friends.

DEATH IN THE FAMILY

Dilly, Belle's older sister, had been in failing health for sometime, so Marilda had moved her into the Osborne household. Dilly had dementia and had to be watched like a toddler. One day Bib and Marilda were going to the grocery store. Marilda had asked her good friend Lou Brown to come and sit with her mother until they came home from the store. They waited for Lou but she never came, so they decided to go on and leave her mother with the children. When they had walked down the road a piece they met Lou. They talked awhile and Lou came on to the house to stay with Dilly. When she got to the porch Dilly was swinging and said, "How come you didn't come to stay? You know Mommy (speaking of her daughter) had to go to the store."

Lou said, "Dilly, I had to help Belle before I could get here."

Dilly replied, "That old Belle Neal! Is she still livin'?"

Dilly had not only lost her mind, but her body was failing also. In June 1951 she passed away. Many people came to the wake and there was much crying and sadness. Dilly's sisters, Belle and Marth, came and were standing out on the porch. Belle looked at Marth and said, "Well, Sister Marth, Sister Dilly is in heaven and that's something to shout about." They shouted and sang till they could be heard all over the holler. Their sister had gone home and they planned to meet her some day. The funeral was set for the next day and the burial would be in the Holcomb Cemetery. They held the service at the Lilly # 11 schoolhouse and then went to the cemetery.

Cordelia was buried in a row that had been designated for Dilly's family. They laid her next to her husband John and three little babies of Bib and Marilda who had died in infancy. Belle was born in May and died in May. Her sister Cordelia was born in June and died in June. Belle and George would rest in a row below Dilly.

MINE EXPLOSION

One warm day in March, Belle and George were sitting out on their front porch just soaking up the sunshine. The peacefulness of the day was shattered when they heard three long blasts at the mines. Belle and George both looked over the mountain where the mines were. Belle told George, "That's a signal for a cave-in! I think they will need all the help they can get, so I'd better go down." George never said a word because he knew that Belle would do as she pleased.

She went into the kitchen and placed her doctor's bag on the table. She checked to see what she had packed and what she would need. She had a large bundle of clean rags but she added another and checked to see if her scissors and cotton were inside. She put a jar of homemade salve in the side of the bag along with several herbs that she might need. She stopped to think what she could use on injuries. She packed a jar of blackberry tea that was good for hemorrhaging, her new stethoscope and a drinking cup for herself. She almost forgot the rubbing alcohol. When she had packed everything she would need, she hollered out to George and told him to saddle Old Boss. She remembered to get herself a coat and some gloves. When she came out onto the porch, George was holding the horse near the steps.

Belle tied her bag on and hoisted herself up on the horse, "You know where to find me, George, if the need arises." George shook his head yes and Belle headed toward the mines. She took a shortcut by way of a logging road and cut through the cherry orchard that belonged to her brother-in-law, John Neal. She dropped down onto Route 16 just below the coal tipple.

Belle stopped a young man with coal dust on his face as he went by leading his mule. "Can you tell me what happened here young man? Are there miners trapped?"

He reluctantly stopped, "Yes, 14 men in two different crews appear to be trapped. Jim Cottrell and I were near the mouth, working with our mules; the blast threw us both toward the outside. We were able to run and save ourselves and our animals."

"Well, I've come to tend the sick. Where do I need to be?"

"I believe I'd go up to the mine office and inquire there. I'm sure they'll be glad to have your help."

When she got close to the mine office she could see groups of people standing around everywhere. Everything seemed to be moving slowly, like in a dream, and no one seemed to know what to do. She rushed to get closer to the door and she saw the little Chinese woman that she had helped deliver her baby some time ago. She went up to the weeping woman and tried to talk with her. She just shook her head that she did not understand and one of her older children talked for her. They had heard the blast, and knowing that their father was in the mines, they rushed over, as every one else did, to find out the news.

Belle looked at the grieving woman, holding the newborn child, and at all the children, none with a winter coat. She told them to go home and she would bring them word when she found out. "These children are going to be cold and hungry. It's best to take them home."

The Chinese woman did not want to leave but she could see that Belle was right, so they went down the road toward home.

Belle finally got to talk with the man at the office and he had no news to tell. They were waiting for the dust to settle and then they planned to send in a crew of workers. Belle asked him if she could make some coffee on his potbelly stove and give it to people.

He told her it would be all right and Belle set to work. She cleaned the big tin coffee pot and filled it with fresh water and grounds. When it was ready she carried the pot around to those who had cups. Most people seemed grateful, knowing that the wait was going to be long and cold!

Belle stayed the night, mixing about in the crowd. Morning came in cold and clear with people huddled together to avoid the chilling air.

They were all hungry, cold and apprehensive. Belle went to the mine office and again made pots of hot coffee to share with the families.

Toward noon some people who worked in the town of Clay came to distribute some sandwiches and drinks. When a mining tragedy happened, it affected the whole area. If one of their own was not in the mines, they knew someone who was inside. The trapped miners were on everyone's mind. Were they alive? Were some hurt and suffering? Could they hold out until help could come?

The crowd began to shift and the mining superintendent stepped up on a table near the mine office and waited until it was quiet. Then he began to tell them about the miners.

"I have been down to the mines and back to the area of the blast. The dust is settling now and we have men who are now slowly removing the wall. At this time, I cannot say if there are any survivors, but I am remaining optimistic. We will not give up until we have found our men." At that, the crowd began to clap and the people seemed to be more relieved, knowing that at least something was being done. They stood around in small groups talking in hushed tones the entire day; the sky was gray and cloudy like their hearts. Some of the miners' wives had come with no warm clothing. The vacant looks on their faces said that they had little hope, for they had lived through these events before.

The life of a coal miner was a hard one and the life of the miner's wife was no better. They lived in company houses that were poorly made with no conveniences—usually having to carry water a long distance from a community well, no inside plumbing, barely enough furniture to fill the dilapidated homes. Living in a mining camp was harsh, with no form of sanitation and no medical aid. Foreigners had life harder than most. Local people did not like to socialize with the Chinese and especially the Negroes. Segregation was a way of life in the 1940s. There was usually a street for blacks and one for foreigners in the coal camps. Belle looked around at the crowd and saw the pain on the faces of all—the blacks, the Chinese, the Italians and the local people. She knew they were all struggling to accept the situation.

Belle had now been here nearly twenty-four hours. She was beginning to wear down and she could see that many others were just as tired as she. The last word that they had heard from the mines was that they believed they were nearing the last of the cave-in. Hope was still high. People wanted to be here if and when they brought the men out, so they stayed. Belle had washed her face and hands and combed her hair. Then she got out her canvas coat with a hood on it, wrapped herself in the warm coat and put on her gloves. She walked among the people and tried to assure them that they would find the miners soon. She kept making coffee and kept an ear toward the mine. Around four o'clock that evening, someone from the mines came running and said that they had reached the first miners. They heard one long blast—the signal for some survivors. People ran toward the mines hoping to see their loved one. Belle stopped long enough to grab her doctor's bag. She was at the mine when they brought out the second miner. The first was lying on a stretcher and they placed the next man by him. Both were alert and seemed to be in fair condition.

Belle worked her way through the crowd and kneeled down to see if they needed medical attention. They first man had a cut on his hand and it had been wrapped in a dirty handkerchief. Belle moved on to the next and saw that he had a large cut on his head and was holding his arm toward his chest. "Is your arm broken?" she asked when she could get close enough for him to hear. He shook his head yes, but was too exhausted to speak.

Belle took charge because no one else did. She asked the people to step back and give them some air. She sent two men to bring fresh water. When she had the sleeve cut from the miner's arm, she felt for the broken bone and set it quickly before the man knew what was happening. She wrapped the arm in clean rags and someone brought her two strips of wood with which she made a splint. When she had finished, she laid the arm upon the man's chest. She mixed an herb tea with hot water from the office. She knew the tea would alleviate the pain and she fed it to him in spoonfuls.

When Belle had done all she could, she wrapped him in a blanket that someone handed her and she moved on to the next man who had been brought out. He was unconscious so she checked his pupils and then used her stethoscope to see if he was breathing. She continued to examine him for injuries and found a large cut on his upper arm. The blood had congealed and dried, leaving the shirt stuck to the wound. She asked for some warm water and someone came back quickly with a bucket. They brought a pan, poured the water in and handed it to Belle. She gently washed the wound and could see that it was going to need stitches.

Belle worked quickly, knowing that it was best to sew the wound while he was unconscious. She took out her black silk thread and swiftly had the needle ready, but first she dipped it in alcohol. She stitched the cut as best she could in the poor light. She then applied some ointment and wrapped it with a clean bandage. Someone who knew the man knelt by him and Belle went back to the first man. He was awake and alert.

She checked his hand and knew he could wait on mending so she cleaned the cut and wrapped it with clean bandages. Someone brought more blankets and she left him as someone was wrapping him up. Two more men were brought out and Belle moved in.

Someone hollered loudly, "Let the granny woman through. She is taking care of the injured." The crowd parted and Belle came through carrying her doctor's bag. She knelt down by one miner and reached for a clean wet rag that someone handed to her. She could find no injuries on the man. She gently washed the black from his face and he groaned but was not fully alert. Someone came by with a blanket and she moved on. The last man they brought out was bleeding heavily. He had been under a pile of slat and it had crushed his pelvis.

Belle knew that she could not help him, but she tried anyway. Unknown hands were there to give her items she needed and another blanket. Belle tried to stop the bleeding by packing the wound with rags, and then she quoted the verse from the Bible that helped stop blood. She covered him with the blanket, passed her hand over his face, placed a drop of oil on his forehead and whispered these words before she stood, "Mark 6:13—anointed with oil many that were sick and healed them." Belle stood up and whispered to herself, "I will leave him in God's hands."

Belle had been so busy that she had not realized that night had fallen once again. Carbine lights were shining all around and fires were built in fifty-gallon drums. Belle had not eaten through the day but she had slipped away once for a cup of coffee at the mine office. She stretched to relieve her throbbing back muscles and realized how hungry she was. Someone passed by and handed her a sandwich as they were doing for all the workers. She took time for a quick bite and then the whistle blew again as they brought more miners out.

Belle moved forward to the new group of men and began an exam to see which ones needed to be treated first. The first man was struggling for breath—he had been trapped inside so long without fresh air. She dropped her head to his chest to check his breathing and then again with her new stethoscope. He seemed to have some fluid on his lungs and his heart was beating too fast. She made a blanket into a pillow and placed it beneath his head. She knew there was little else she could do for him. They had him out in the fresh air and that should improve his breathing. Again she was handed a blanket and she wrapped it around him.

They had just brought two more miners out and Belle moved over to where they lay. She examined the first miner, but he was gone. He was the husband of the Chinese woman that she had sent home with her children.

Belle dropped her head in defeat, for she knew that as hard as things were in the coal camp, that woman would have it even harder without a husband and father for her children. She would have to leave the company house and travel on to a new location. Belle was thinking that she needed to get to the family before someone else did. She stood up and looked all around. The scene appeared foggy, the location seemed dreary and everyone was moving as if in a dream. Voices could be heard but they all seemed to blend together. Belle sensed that she was going to faint and she quickly sat down on the damp, cold ground and put her head between her knees. That helped and she was told that the second crew was being brought out. Most were dead. Families who had kept a vigil through the long days and nights now cried and mourned for their lost love ones. When all of the men had been rescued and the dead lay together, Belle gathered her doctor's bag and found her horse. Then she headed for the home of the Chinese miner.

When she was almost to the house, she could see the woman and the children standing on the porch looking bleak and sad. For a while all she could see were their sad eyes; they knew before she said anything that the news was not good. She took the baby in her arms and consoled the rest as much as she could. She spoke to the mother through the son and learned that they had relatives in Kanawha County where they could go. Belle told them that she would come back and help them pack their few belongings after she got some rest. She hated to leave them, but she was exhausted and hungry, so she lit her lantern and rode up the mountain path toward home.

The mining disaster was all that was talked about in Bickmore. The section where the disaster had occurred would be shut down for a while, meaning the miners would lose work. It took about two weeks to have all the funerals. Some days people attended services and burials all day long. There was a hush across the neighborhood— no loud talking or complaining, just sad faces and open graves as the dead were laid to rest.

Belle went back and helped the Chinese woman with what she owned: an old mattress and frame, a few pots and pans, and some ragged quilts that the children made into beds. A man who knew them brought a horse and wagon up to the steps and Belle helped him load their meager supplies. Then the mother and children said their goodbyes and Belle could tell by the woman's face that she was thankful to Belle, even though she could not say the words in English. Belle just patted her arm and waved to them until they were out of sight.

Then Belle went inside and scrubbed the rooms with a bucket of hot water, swept up the debris that was scattered around, closed the door and headed home.

Days flew by, time moved on, and so did the people. Many families moved into the coal camps at Rock Cut or Red Row. Unnamed rows of houses were quickly built and occupied and the cycle began again. People were married, babies were born and the old and sick died. Mountain people lived each day the best they knew how, at times just existing. Most did not complain about their situation. They were glad to have a home and a place to raise their families.

A FIGHT WITH A PIG

One day in early spring John L. Brown came to visit his cousin Belle. John was a veterinarian and he and Belle liked to discuss medical situations. They had a good long visit and sat on the porch and drank some coffee. When they had caught up on the doings of the family and their medical endeavors, John said he should be on his way home.

Belle said, "John, I have a whole parcel of piglets and I would like to give you one to raise for this winter's food." John agreed and appreciated the offer. Belle said, "We will have to go and take it from its Momma." Hogs ran freely in the woods and grew large tusks. The old mother looked vicious and mean; and most people shied away from her. But Belle waded right on in as the mother was ready to attack.

John yelled, "Belle! That hog is going to eat you up!"

Belle kept walking and as she picked up a piglet the old mother charged. Belle stood her ground and landed a booted foot into the center of the old hog's head. The hog backed off squealing and grunting. Belle came out holding the pig by the two back legs. She tied them with jute and handed the pig to John. He just shook his head and said to himself, "I should know better than to worry. Belle lets nothing stop her when she has a notion on her mind."

In the summer of 1948, John was surveying some land in Leatherwood and Bickmore. He walked over the mountain and down to the community well at Red Row. He was hot and tired on this summer day. As he sat down to rest by the well he died, apparently of a heart attack.

LIFE ON THE FARM

"Today looks like a good day to churn," Belle thought, as she looked out the window early one morning. She had just milked her cow and was straining the milk. She got out her butter churn, poured the milk and began to work the dasher. She had already scalded her pans and the churn, and was hoping for three or four pounds of fresh butter. It was a tiring job that she was always glad to finish. Belle disliked being confined in one spot for long. She checked the milk and dashed harder.

As she sat there alone in her kitchen, she let her mind wander. She was thinking how good God had been to her through the years when she realized that she did not have many years left. Belle wished that she had accomplished more in her time, but she was thankful that God had spared her this long. She was blessed to have been given a talent to assist in childbirth and care for the sick.

She had forgotten about time and could feel the butter coming in the churn. She looked and decided that it was strong enough to make into molds. She removed the white, creamy butter with a wooden paddle. She molded four dishes and covered them with a clean piece of cheesecloth. When she had wrapped them all and stored them in the cellar, she strained the buttermilk and added a pinch of salt. She stopped to have a taste and thought, as she drank, that nothing tasted as good as fresh churned buttermilk—it was one of her favorites.

She placed the remainder of the milk in a big brown crock pitcher and after covering it, she took it to the cellar and placed it by the butter. Homer would be over soon to get some butter for Marilda; she was glad that the chore was done until next week.

"Today looks like a good day to harvest some more herbs," she thought. After she tidied up the kitchen, she got down her big feed sack with the strap she had sewn on so she could carry it over her shoulder. She had made a mental note as to what she would look for today. Pennyroyal was first. While not plentiful in this area, she had seen some and wanted it to make a good insect repellent. There was nothing better in her opinion. Rats bane or pipsissewa was used for the kidneys. She was sure there was some growing on the hillside past her her garden. Boiled and strained it would be made into a warm tea.

One thing she really wanted to harvest was Indian tobacco. She liked to dig it up by the roots and hang it on her porch to dry in pods. It had many medicinal uses, but Belle liked to use it as a smoke for her pipe.

Belle walked a little slower now. Climbing the hills was harder, especially with arthritis in her knees. She was thinking that she would mix herself a good tonic for the stiffness when she got home. Belle was so used to taking care of everyone else that she often forgot to take care of herself. But 'these old bones,' as she now thought of herself, would remind her often.

Belle walked on around the ridge using a walking stick for support. As she looked down, she identified burdock. She had nearly stepped on it! She kneeled to gather a little of the leaf and was thinking that she could use it as a purifier for blood. Belle came to a spot in the woods that had fewer trees and she looked up to see the sun shedding its bright rays through the leaves, illuminating the forest floor. She stooped when she saw a purple lady slipper peeping through the leaves. She bent down to examine the fragile plant, touching it lightly and removing the dead leaves that covered the flower.

People often stopped by Belle's home to ask advice on some herb or for a cure for an illness. People could go into the woods as she did and make their own medicine, but Belle usually had a little of everything stored away. She loved to make tonics and teas or ointments and poultices. She liked to treat the sick and she had a soothing hand.

As Belle walked back down the hill toward her cabin she thought about how much she liked going into the woods and gathering her own herbs. She closed her eyes and recalled a verse from the Bible that she had often thought about: "Beloved I have given you every herb, every seed which is upon the face of the earth."—Genesis 1:29-30. Belle felt humbled that God had used her to heal the sick. She could not have been given a greater blessing.

George and Belle made it through another winter. Belle had a spinning wheel and she spun wool that winter to make rugs. George sat near the fire and Belle sat in her rocker and kept her hands busy. They tuned the radio to a comedy, preaching, or the news of the world.

Nothing essential happened that winter, as they remained snowbound most of the time. They kept their cabin warm with coal in the fireplace and the cook stove. When the weather warmed, Belle was hungry for some company, so she wrapped herself in warm clothes, pulled on the old rubber boots and set out to visit her niece Marilda.

The weather still had a sting when it hit her face but the clean, crisp air renewed her body. She dropped down over the hill on a path that took her to the houses. She stopped first at Okey's house to see how their latest addition was doing. Grace, born in August last year, was a happy, contented baby with curly black hair. She visited awhile and bounced the baby on her knee as she talked. Soon she thought she should move on so she could get home before dark.

When she got to Marilda's house, it was quieter than usual. The children were in school and the new baby, Mary, was sleeping. Marilda had certainly had a hard time getting Little Mary into the world, Belle thought. She had to be rushed to a hospital in Charleston, where they delivered Mary. Marilda had been having seizures and they were afraid for the unborn child, but both were healthy now.

Soon they could hear the older children coming up the road from school. Forest, Homer and Ruth came into the house yelling at each other. Ruth was almost in tears. She said that she that she had slipped and fallen on the way to school and Homer and Forest just left her. A woman who lived nearby heard her crying, took her in and dried her clothes near the fire. On the return trip the boys had stopped to take her home.

Ruth said that no matter what happened they always made her carry home the tin bucket they used for their lunch. Marilda scolded the boys. While Ruth had their attention she thought she would tell her about another event. Last week Marilda had fixed their sandwiches with store-bought bread. Ruth was so happy to have the store-bought bread she would hide it behind her back after she took a bite. Mostly she was afraid the other children would ask for a bite. While the bread was behind her back, a mean, old rooster that wandered the schoolyard reached up and took her sandwich. She cried the rest of the day. Marilda and Belle sympathized with her but could not keep from laughing.

SPRING REVIVAL

After a good revival in spring, the church would always have a big baptizing. People came from every community to witness the event. It did not matter what the denomination, they all came to share the big dinner after the baptizing and have a visit with neighbors.

They had gathered at a large hole of water at the mouth of Sycamore Creek. The people sat around; some were talking, some were singing and some were just being quiet, knowing that this was a sacred time. The men who were to be baptized stood together and the women and girls stood in a circle with white sheets wrapped around them from head to toe. They took turns placing pebbles in the hems of their sheets so that the covering would not float when they went under. The two preachers waded out into the water and checked to see if there was any sharp debris that would hurt someone. While they were wading they would take handfuls of water and throw it upon their clothes to adapt to the chilly water.

The people who were going to sing gathered in a circle and began to sing *Shall We Gather at the River*, *Amazing Grace* and *I Shall Not Be Moved*. The men went first and the preachers dedicated the new converts to God as they went under and came up, cleansed and renewed. Then the women came out one by one, and they too were washed in the cleansing blood of Jesus. When the baptism was over, the crowd moved to the church for a picnic on the grounds. A group of men who had brought instruments played gospel songs and everyone joined in. The young men and women walked up and down the road flirting.

The preacher announced that the service was about to end as the sun was dipping behind the mountain.

The darkness came quicker in the valleys and people who walked needed to leave now to get home before full darkness. Families gathered their children and all bowed their heads as the preacher ended with a prayer.

Everyone packed away the remains of the picnic. You could hear the rattle of the old wagons, the motors of the old cars and the sound of children laughing as they all headed for home. The preacher closed the church doors and headed for his own home, thankful for the wonderful day.

AUNT BELLE TO THE RESCUE

Ann was playing by herself one day. She had a bottle of pop and tried to get it open by driving a nail in the lid. The bottle exploded and drove glass shards into her leg. When Marilda saw the damage, she took Ann to Belle's house. Aunt Belle sat her on the kitchen table, cleaned it and pulled the glass out. When it was clean, she took a little of her Mickey Twist tobacco and placed it over the cut to draw out any infection. She wrapped it with a clean cloth; the wound healed nicely.

About twenty years later, a knot appeared on her leg so Ann went to visit the doctor. He lanced the leg and removed a tobacco stem about an inch long. Ann recalled when Belle had treated the leg with tobacco, and marveled at how it had healed.

WRESTLING WITH A PANTHER

Neighbors of George and Belle and Belle were fond of them. As they got older, neighbors helped them. When one neighbor had a hog killing, he told George and Belle to come to his house. They went and when the killing was done, Belle and George got a quarter of the meat. It was placed in a feed sack and George carried it on his back. They had to walk through the woods as it was getting dark. Belle led the way with a lantern and George carried the ham. George could not turn around with the load he carried, but he thought there was something behind him. He yelled at Belle and told her to look behind him. She looked and sure enough, there was a panther following them. Belle took the sack and she and George walked on toward home.

When they were closer to home, Belle turned quickly and hit the cat in the head with the ham. The panther was so stunned that it ran into the woods. When George told of the event later, he would say, "Well, Belle just took the sack and went on home."

EPIDEMIC!!!

One fall season the children in the area began to miss school with a sickness that hit entire families. Soon the Board of Education realized they had an epidemic on their hands. Everyone was on alert, not knowing what caused the disease or how to treat it. None had died yet, but it continued to strike whole families.

Belle recognized the illness by its symptoms; she feared it was typhoid fever. The board sent word to all the families in the area to remain in their homes until the disease was determined. If the disease was as Belle expected, untreated it could wipe out a whole family. Belle had seen this before and she knew the procedure it would take to stop it. When she was younger she helped her father and her uncle treat typhoid. The first symptoms were profuse sweating, rose-colored spots on the lower chest, fevers raging to 104 degrees and a distended, painful abdomen.

People were confined to small areas, especially during the winter months, as the disease was highly contagious. Later symptoms were diarrhea and intestinal hemorrhage that usually lasted three weeks to a month. If the lower intestines perforated, it would cause pain and sometimes even death. Typhoid was a disease that would spread very fast, especially in a community with little medical treatment.

Belle began to work with her neighbors. She went from house to house in her community and treated those in need until the disease played out. No one succumbed to the fever this time. It was necessary to keep vigils over the patients, providing a soft diet until the intestines were healed. But people needed to be educated on better sewer systems and clean water sources. School vaccines became mandatory and in the following years, the school board's ruling on vaccines eradicated many childhood illnesses.

Typhoid fever was brought on by unclean water, insects carrying disease from open sewers, poor sanitation, unhealthy diets and poor hygiene—especially in winter. Plagues, such as lice, scabies, the itch, and many other pests are, still to this day, undefeated in schools.

Belle became discouraged when she worked in her neighbors' homes where the illness was largely due to poor hygiene. She and her niece Marlida were summoned to a house at Glen to deliver a baby. Belle had been there many times, and each time she was forced to explain the need for better cleaning habits to the resident. Each time she returned, she found living conditions just as bad, if not worse, as before. When she and Marilda arrived, they found dirty dishes, garbage and food items strung around the kitchen. Someone had left the door open and chickens were walking across the table. Belle and Marilda set in to cleaning the kitchen since they would be there for a number of days and would not eat until the kitchen was cleaned.

When the child was born and everything taken care of, Belle sat down to have a heart to heart talk with the mother. "Ella, if you do not get in the habit of keeping a cleaner house, I will not come back to bring anymore babies into this hovel. You always tell me that things will be better and instead they are worse! Your children are sick and poorly because of the pigpen in which they live. Sleeping in dirty beds, eating in a dirty kitchen and breathing the dirty air…if you do not clean this place up you will be burying your children with some type of disease. I will not come back to this house to deliver anymore babies for you until I see some improvement."

This made the woman cry and again she promised to do better, but Belle doubted it. She made a promise to herself if she came back again and waded through filth, she would walk right back out the door.

MAN MEETS GHOST

Belle's nephew, Okey Neal, and her nephew by marriage, Bib Osborne, worked at the Ward Mines about three miles from their home. They carried their lunch pails and wore their hardhats with the carbide lights attached as they walked to the mines. When they worked the evening shift, they walked home using their carbide lights to see the way. One such night, they had just turned off of Route 16 and onto Osborne Fork, where they had to ford the creek that crisscrossed the road several times. When they neared the water hole where the women did laundry, the men came around a curve in the road and were surprised to see a light coming toward them. They said nothing and continued to watch the light. When it passed them, they both looked on in wonder, seeing a man walk by them without a head. They were honest men who would not fabricate such a story and they told it to their families.

Through the years many other strange episodes occurred, such as a shrill holler at night from the woods that would pierce the stillness and awaken the residents of the little hollow. When Marilda and her siblings were young, they were just sitting down for a meal when they heard someone running around the house and singing a song that was popular at the time about the sinking of the Titanic. They all assumed that it was their only brother, Okey. They were not alarmed until they realized Okey was not home yet. Who knows or can say if such things happen; it is just a brief instance witnessed by a few and they felt it was real to them.

Belle told another story of a night when George was working the mines. She went to bed and was asleep when she heard George call her. She got up, lit the lantern and walked out to the gate in her yard, but there was no one there. She shook her head and went back to bed. The next night she again heard George calling her. She went to the gate and this time George was there. He was sick and had left the mines early. Belle didn't question these events. There were things that could not be explained and this was one of them.

A REMEDY FOR BELLE

It was blackberry winter here, the last of May and the 1st week of June, when the berries bloomed each year. An old wives' tale said that if it rained on the bloom on the third day of June, the berries would not produce well and the fruit would be bitter. Belle thought about the berries and rubbed her chapped hands. They were rough and sore today. She remembered that she had heard of an herbal remedy to soothe the skin. She went to get some of the dried rose petals that she had stored from last year.

She crushed a few, added them to hot water and let them steep for a while. Then she took some olive oil and a small amount of lanolin and mixed them together. She then strained the rose water, adding a few more products that she knew would help in healing, and added it to the mixture, blending with her hands. When it reached the stage that was thick enough to rub, she placed the mixture into small glass jars and labeled them for use. She relished in the soothing cream as she rubbed the solution into her hands. She loved the scent of fresh roses. She thought she would make some for gifts when she had time.

At times Belle had a few days when she wasn't called on to doctor; she was at a loss when she was idle. For as long as she could remember, she was busy living, doctoring and caring for others—it seemed strange when she had time for herself. She worked in her garden, and cooked and cared for her family, but her love of doctoring was never far from her mind. As she was weeding her garden she checked the cucumber vines to see if she would have enough for a churn of pickles. It looked like she could gather a basketful of the young and tender ones and work up a batch tomorrow if the signs were right for pickling. She gathered a few yellow squash to cook for supper.

She checked to see that she had enough salt, vinegar and spices for the pickles. When she had fixed a meal, she gathered the cucumbers and the items she would use and placed them on the table. She went to the cellar and brought in a 5-gallon churn. She scalded the churn and left it with the rest of the items. She would get an early start in the morning before the sun heated the house.

Belle went to check on her strawberry patch to see if the plants were bearing well. She and her sisters, Cordelia and Martha, had ordered plants from a seed catalog last year and had been tenderly caring for them. This year they should yield a good crop. They were now in full bloom. Belle lifted one plant and found some strawberries that were still green; she should have her first batch in a week or two. Secretly, she wanted to have a better harvest than her sisters, but she would not tell them so. The proof was in the crop and she would take some to show them! It was summertime again and all of God's creation was bringing forth fruit. Belle tried to keep a close watch on her garden, for if she was called away for doctoring she might lose a crop that she had been waiting for.

FAMILY REUNION

Belle and George walked to the post office at Bickmore near the last of June. They spent time talking with townsfolk around the post office, as they wanted to rest before they took the long walk home. One of Belle's nephews told them about a family reunion that Hal had planned. It was on the fourth of July and they were to spread the news to all the family. Belle was hesitant to go because she didn't like some of her distant relatives. She told her nephew Ike that she would consider the invitation. In the end Belle and George decided to go.

Hal sent word that he would come and get them. Belle said no; they would walk. They were a little late getting to the reunion and most of the people had already arrived. Everyone who knew Belle noticed them as they were coming in. Belle was wearing one of her clean housedresses and a feed sack apron. On her feet were a pair of high top work boots; her hair was pulled back in a severely tight bun.

When Belle walked up on the porch she marched over to a woman of whom she did not approve. Belle pointed a finger at the Hedrick woman, and in a loud voice, she said, "There is the woman who mistreated my mother." For a minute everyone was quiet and waited to see what the outcome would be. The Hedrick woman knew better than to get in a discussion with Belle, so she thought it wise to remain quiet. Soon people around them began to talk in hushed tones and the moment passed. Belle's mother had been dead for some time, but Belle had been waiting for her opportunity to embarrass the woman. When she was done, she mingled around and talked to relatives. At future family events, relatives would talk to each other about Belle and her outspoken, sometimes rude, comments.

GRANDCHILDREN

It was a beautiful summer evening; George and Belle were sitting on their porch visiting with their children and grandchildren. The air was balmy. It was relaxing to sit and soak up the fresh air, and comforting to know everyone could be idle today and just enjoy the time together. Belle had fixed a dinner of fried chicken and dumplings and they had fed so many that the table had to be spread three times. It wasn't often that they had all of the children and grandchildren together and no one wanted to spoil the day by leaving early. The grandchildren had played hide and seek until dark. Now they were catching fireflies and keeping them in a glass jar. They were laughing and shouting at each other as they darted to see who could catch the most.

It was still light enough to see that the children were being bitten, so Belle went to get her remedy for insect bites. She took her jar of dried basil and poured a small amount into a clean rag. She crushed the basil until it was fine, and then added a small amount of water to form a paste. She took it to her grandchildren and told them to spread the mixture onto their legs and arms.

George was sitting on his mules ear tobacco chair leaning against the wall. He asked Belle what she was doing and she told him that the basil made a good bug repellent. George just shook his head and watched. As they relaxed it would grow quiet for a time and then they would listen to the sounds of the warm night: the frogs, birds, and whippoorwill; the baying of the hounds over the ridge; the blowing of the old horse in the stall; and the faint sound of the evening breeze as it ruffled the leaves on the trees. The children, with joy and innocence of youth, mixed around the porch where their parents sat. As the sun dropped behind the hill, they looked up to a red sky in the west and decided that tomorrow would be a wonderful day.

SCHOOL TIME

It was a wonderful fall day. The leaves were still on the trees, their vibrant colors bright against the clear blue sky. School had started three weeks before and a salesman made a call to Lilly #11 school. He prompted the children to go to their neighbors and sell his product and they would receive a prize. This was real incentive for children who were rarely awarded something material for their work. That possibility caused them to branch out to even the most remote homes seeking sales.

Ruth and her first cousin, Mozelle, daughter of Leslie, decided to go to see their Aunt Belle. Immediately after school they walked to Belle's house and asked her to buy their products. When they arrived, Aunt Belle led them to the kitchen where she had a pan of warm cornbread and fresh homemade butter on the table. She told the girls to fix themselves something to eat. It tasted wonderful; they had not had anything to eat since their sandwiches at noon. They piled the fresh butter on the warm cornbread. It melted and ran down their arms, but they were too satisfied to care.

Belle looked over the item they had for sale. It was Cloverine salve, packaged in small tin cans. It was always a good medicine to have on hand because it was so versatile. It cost 50 cents each or three for a dollar. Belle knew that she could use the the salve, but had to see if she had a dollar. She was able to pay one dollar in change and the girls were pleased.

When the salesman came back to school, Ruth and Mozell each received a small change purse for the tins they had sold.

BELLE COMES OFF THE MOUNTAIN

When Belle looked out her kitchen window early one morning she saw a man guiding a horse, standing on a sled being pulled behind. She did not recognize him but she knew that he was coming for her. She stepped out on her porch and could see that he was a man from Hartland. She spoke before he stepped from the sled. "Howdy Ed, what brings you here so early?"

"Hi Belle, my woman has taken sick and she has been down for about a week this time. She doesn't seem to get any better and the kids and me have done all we can for her. Do you think you could come and see her?"

"Why sure Ed, I can do that. But first tell me what kind of aliments she's had."

"She could be feeling fine and next thing you know, she is having pains so bad she has to lay down. Sometimes that would last about 12 hours, just whirling in pain. Nothing we do seems to help. She might be all right for a day or two and then it starts all over again. She eats very little and she has lost a lot of weight."

"So you think this might be some stomach problem?"

"I cain't rightly say but she has also been vomiting up bile."

"Well, I'll get some things together and go with you. Come in and have a cup of coffee. I was just ready to have breakfast."

Ed tied the horse to a tree near the house and went in and spoke to George and Radar who were at the table.

"Hi George, how you been, I haven't seen you in quite a spell."

"Hello, Ed, I don't get out too much—gettin' too old to travel. I ache all the time now."

Belle went to get her doctor's bag and loaded it with some parsley, dandelion, marshmallow leaf and shave grass in separate glass containers. She knew that she could fix a remedy to purge the body, but she would not mix them together until she saw the patient. She made sure her instruments were cleaned and ready. She made a quick trip to the cellar which yielded some of her "bitters" stored in sealed glass jars. She took an extra change of clothes, a light shawl and some nightclothes. She gave Radar and George orders on things she needed to be done and then she was off.

Ed helped her on the sled and tied her bag behind her.

"It might be a little rough, Belle, but I'll take it slow. Hold on now," he said as they pulled away.

"You take care of the horse and sled Ed, and I'll take care of Belle Neal."

They headed back up the rough road. The sled rocked back and forth and Belle had to hold on tightly until they reached the crossroads at the top of Beechy Ridge road. When they reached the top, Ed let the horse cool down and rest for a while. Marv and Lou's children were playing around the road and they wanted to know where Grandma was going. Katie, Hazel, Paula, Marion and the younger children, Betty and Brady, ran down to see their grandmother.

"I'm going to be gone for a few days. Would you tell Lou and Marv to look in on George and Radar?"

"Yell we will do that. Goodbye, Grandma!" They waved until the sled was out of sight and then they ran home to tell their mother.

Ed drove the sled along the brim of the road when they reached Route 16. They passed several people and many stopped to say hello. Some people on their porches waved as the sled went down the road.

They got to the Elk River and had to wait for a ferry. Belle got off the sled and stretched her legs while they waited. Belle didn't like to ride the ferry, but the other route was much longer. They would have had to go on the north side of the river, follow the railroad tracks, cross the Dundon Bridge above Clay, and go south again through Clay. She didn't say anything to Ed but she would be glad when they were across the river. The ferry operator finally came back and began to load the horses, buggies, and cars. He tied them all down and, at the rear, he tied the sled down. Belle walked over to the side of the ferry and held on to the rail.

When they arrived at the other side of the river, Ed and Belle were the first to get off.

Ed helped Belle on the sled and they went up the road about 500 feet. Then Ed guided the sled up a steep road and to the house where he lived. Belle looked around and could see that many things had been ignored. The dogs had been digging in the yard and the children had left their playthings scattered around. When Belle stepped up onto the porch, the dogs jumped up from their dirty rugs and barked and nipped at her. She gave the two in front a swift kick and they backed down. "Don't mess with me, you scraggly curs," she said, "I'll knock your brains out." She stood her ground and the dogs whimpered and backed down.

She stepped in through the door and everything was in such disarray that it was hard to find a path to walk through. The children were in awe of this sharp-tongued woman. They soon forgot their shyness, though, as Belle took charge. They were glad she had come.

Belle went to see the mother. Belle asked her about her symptoms and looked at her skin, which was ashen. She had dark circles beneath her eyes. Belle examined her stomach and asked where the pain was most severe. It seemed that the pain traveled from her chest and around her shoulder, lodging in the back and remaining sharp until the attack passed, leaving her sore and weak. She said that she could hardly keep any food down and at times, even water came back up.

Belle made her up a fresh bed and told her to rest until she had prepared a meal for the family. Blanche was relieved to have someone to help.

Belle went to the kitchen and took some of the herbs out of her bag. She mixed several that she knew would help purge the woman and get the inflammation out of the system. She poured hot water over the mixture, then added a little honey and a teaspoon of whiskey. She took it in to Blanche and told her to sip it slowly and that it should help her sleep.

Belle went in where the children were and asked the older girls to come and help her fix a hot meal. She got the other children to clean up the house and yard. The girls helped Belle find the makings of a large meal. Belle put water on the stove to boil and ordered the girls to wash up the dishes and clean the kitchen.

Belle peeled potatoes and she put them on the stove to boil. She mixed up a batch of cornbread, hoping it was enough to feed a large starving family. She went into the pantry and found some home-canned beans and opened up enough to fill a big cooker. She placed them on the stove and sent Ed to the smokehouse for a slab of bacon. Belle fried the meat and saved the grease for seasoning.

The girls went to get some fresh buttermilk from their springhouse and set the table. Finally, they all sat down to one of the first hot meals they had eaten in awhile. Belle fixed a plate with mashed potatoes and butter and took the plate to Blanche.

Blanche tried to eat but she was nauseated, so Belle went to the table and ate with the family. When they had finished the meal, Belle sent the boys to bring in water and put the girls to cleaning the kitchen.

While the kids were busy, Belle sat down with Ed to discuss the ailments Blanche had.

"Ed, from her symptoms, I think that Blanche has gallstones. I cannot do much for her. She needs to go to the hospital in Charleston and have surgery to have them removed."

"I was afraid it would need a doctor's surgery, but I don't see how we can pay for that," said Ed.

"You don't have much of a choice," said Belle, "If you don't take her, she could die from the infection and disease that would finally take over."

"I'll go and talk to Blanche and see what she thinks," said Ed.

"Well, I'll stay here a couple of days and help the children around the house," said Belle.

Ed gave her a nod of approval and went to talk with his wife. They finally settled on going to the hospital the next day. Ed had to get someone with a car to take them. Belle stayed a while, but knowing the children were old enough to take care of themselves, she decided to go home. The children thanked her and promised to get word to her about their mother. Belle thanked them. She walked to Clay and hitched a ride across the Dundon Bridge and down the railroad grade, south toward home.

THE PEDDLER

On a brisk March evening Belle went into the house after spending the day outside. The weather cooled down quickly after the sun dropped behind the mountain. Belle knew that spring could not be far behind, as she saw crocus blooming. She had also been seeing robins pecking the ground for two weeks now. But the rain that came near dark was making the holler misty and cold; fog was hanging low, making it difficult to see any distance. She was cleaning up the kitchen after the evening meal when she thought she heard someone calling. She stepped up to the window and could see the outline of a man standing in the road. She opened the door and stood on the porch trying to see who was there. Again, a man's voice said, "Hello, in the house."

Belle stepped out unto the steps and yelled back, "Yes, who's there?"

"Ma'am, I'm a traveler passing through. Could I rest on your porch for a spell?"

"Come on in, and I'll get you something to drink."

He waddled across the foot log and she could see he was carrying a huge pack on his back that rattled with every step he took. He removed the burden as soon as he got out of the rain. He had a strip of rope hanging from his neck, like a harness, that held a bedroll hanging down his back beneath the heavy pack. When he dropped the pack he sighed with relief to be done with the weight.

Belle said, "Go on and sit down there and I'll fix you some food. It looks like you haven't eaten a good meal in awhile."

George was sitting near the fire listening to the radio and Radar was outside tending the animals. Belle fixed a plate and poured a cup of hot coffee. When she got out to the porch, the man was sitting on the floor with his back resting against the wall and he had his eyes closed.

Belle spoke, "Here, now, is a bite to eat and some hot coffee that will warm you up."

She placed the food beside him and sat down to talk to him as he ate. "What brings you here, mister?"

"I'm just traveling through. I peddle things to people far from towns. I've got about anything you would need in that pack."

He motioned to the bundle he had taken off.

"I'm not familiar with this area, but I am taking the back roads, knowing that people would be living somewhere along the roads."

"Looks to me like you could get yourself killed traveling where you don't know the way or how of people."

"Yes, I am in danger at times, but most people are friendly and helpful as long as I don't overstep my bounds. Besides I came from across the water where we fought for our lives. Many of us fled the country and came to America. I am a Jew and we have lived in constant danger since the beginning of the war because the Germans wanted to kill us all."

"Well, you're safe here as long as you don't steal or try to hurt us."

"I thank you; I did not get your name. My name is Leendert," he said as he held out his hand to shake Belle's.

"I'm Belle; it's good to meet ye," she said as she held out her hand and grasped his with a firm grip.

"Ms. Belle, would you mind if I bed down on your porch here for the night? I could at least have a roof over my head to avoid the rain."

"I guess you could. I'll fix you some breakfast in the morning before you leave."

"Thank you Mam and good night."

"Good night," she said as she went inside.

When morning came Belle could see the man covered and lying still on the porch. She began to fix a hot breakfast and decided to let him sleep until it was ready. When she went outside to wake the man, he was tossing and turning on his bedroll and talking out of his head. She kneeled down to see if he was running a fever and found that he was burning up. She leaned down and listened to his chest; his breaths were raspy. She called for Radar to help her get him inside.

While Radar went to get a mattress for him to lie on, Belle began to assess his condition. It looked like lung fever. She had to remove his damp clothes and get him in bed. She removed his shoes and socks and then went for some bed linens and made up the mattress near the fire. Radar lifted the man into the bed and Belle placed two pillows behind his head to keep him in a reclining position. If it was pneumonia, he could not lay flat.

She got some tepid water and wiped his face and hands. She rubbed some cloverine salve on his feet and put some wool socks over that. She fixed some mullein leaf tea and placed it in small bowls around in the room to help open the peddler's congested lungs. She also fixed him a hot tea and spooned it in his mouth, hoping to bring down the fever. He finally became quiet and slept.

Belle took the time to eat her own breakfast and told George what the man had told her the night before. The man remained in a near unconscious state for three days as Belle nursed him back to health. On the forth day he became more alert and wanted to talk as he rested.

"I'm so sorry to bring you distress, Ms. Belle. I had no idea I was that sick, but I am thankful that it was here that I came. You have the hands of angels."

"I'm no angel," she said and laughed, "just ask anyone around here."

"To me you are anyway. I will not forget and I hope to leave tomorrow. I do not want to be a burden."

"Stay until you feel better. I would not want to send anyone out sick."

They talked and she learned his story as she sat by the window doing some handwork on a quilt. When World War II started, he and his family lived in a village in France. Hitler began to arrest and persecute all Jews, and even though he tried to keep his family hidden, they, along with most of his neighbors, were taken captive and put into train cars and shipped away to prisons. He tried to keep his wife

and three children with him as they moved across the country by
railroad. One day the Germans separated the men from the women
and children. He never saw his family again. When the war was over,
he worked his way to America by hiring out on a ship. He came and
started the business he now had and was walking his way through
the country. He had no desire to return to his own country because
there were too many memories of sadness there.

Belle had never talked with anyone from another country and
she felt real pity for him. How hard it would be to go on living when
you never knew if your family was dead or alive. He stayed another
night and before bedtime he thanked them and told them that he
would be leaving in the morning and wanted to pay them for his stay.
Both George and Belle refused to accept payment and he thanked
them for saving his life. The next morning Belle awakened and slowly
slipped out of bed. When she walked by the fireplace she realized
that the guest had already left. On his bed were a small package and
a note, which read:

> *Ms. Belle, I can never thank you enough for saving my life.
> God truly sent me your way and I will always be thankful to
> you. I know you will not accept money, but I want to give you
> something and so you should look in the little package on the
> bed. Think of me when you are sewing.*
> *Warm regards: Leendert*

Belle picked up the package and looked inside. There was a gold
thimble, a small pair of gold scissors, and some spools of thread.
Belle admired them and put them on the fireboard mantle until
she cooked breakfast. Belle kept a lot of her treasured items on the
mantle, or fireboard as she called it.

She stepped out onto the porch and she could see Leendert
walking slowly up the rough road, weighted down with his wares.
She stood on the steps and yelled at him. He turned and waved and
Belle did the same.

MINE STRIKE!

In the early 1950s, after a walk to the post office at Bickmore, as Belle was visiting with friends, she heard about the Widen mine strike. Everyone knew someone who worked the mines or was related to a miner. The Widen mine was the single largest employer in Clay County. Clay County. Belle's cousin Joe asked her to Widen to help deliver his baby. The doctors and three women including Joe's wife had left the area when the strike became dangerous.

Belle accepted the offer and went home to pack a few items in her doctor's bag. She added some clothing and a loaded pistol. Belle knew that tempers were were short; violence could likely accelerate over minor events.

Most of the people in the area were in sympathy with the miners. JG Bradley founded the town of Widen when he was a fresh graduate from Harvard. It was a non-union mine but Bradley took very good care of his workers. The self-sufficient town of Widen was a marvel; the whole town had been built with the interest of the workers at heart. The homes were constructed better than most other mining homes. Cheerfully painted red, each one had a picket fence and its own yard. A bank, a theater, schools, churches, a hospital, a country club, a baseball diamond and a car dealership were among the conveniences in the town. The history of the town is published in the archives of Cornell University, stating that no other town in America was as self-sufficient.

The Widen mine was twenty miles from any other town, so it was forced to be independent to survive. Many of the families in Widen worked three generations in the mines at one time. The older men worked as long as their bodies held out. The son worked to care for a large family and his sons went to work alongside of their father. It was a way of life for those who dwelled here; mining was in their blood and in their people. JG Bradley respected his people, paying his workers on a union scale, and did not expect the union to attack his domain. Two earlier strikes in the 30s and 40s did not affect much change in Widen.

But in 1952, union men moved in, surrounding the town of Widen from every mountain peak. They looked down on the town and fired shots at random. Baldwin-Felts or Pinkerton type detectives came to put pressure on the owners with their own means of warfare. Mine sentries were put on guard to protect their turf, and state police were present to keep peace. Guns became a popular part of attire in Widen. Most walked softly, but wanted to be prepared when violence arose.

Ruth and Lloyd owned the local car dealership. They had to check in daily as they came into town to work. Their home was on the mountain leading to Dille. Lloyd told Ruth if she heard gunfire when she was at home to quickly notify the law. Daily tempers flared; hostility and stress were apparent everywhere. During one episode, a gun battle played out near the Butcher home with Ruth and her family inside. The detectives always maintained that they lost none of their own to gunfire, but Ruth saw them carrying a man, apparently dead, from the woods in the cover of darkness.

Townspeople hunkered down for 16 months. They never thought of leaving, because this was their home; they felt they could outlast the union men. But they walked with care as they went about their lives. A Widen woman named Opal was on her way to the company store when she heard several men arguing by the tipple. She quickly moved on to the store and away from the fight that was brewing. She had not been in the store long when shots were heard. Several men entered the store carrying a man with a shotgun wound. They laid his limp body out on the pool table. He was bleeding profusely and he was practically dead on arrival.

Opal, along with several others, was summoned to testify in court about this event. People tried to go on with their normal lives, but were forced to dodge bullets as the days passed. The thugs had created their own law. One man received prison time for the death of the man shot at the tipple. Bradley never backed down, and union men began to back off after events continued to cost lives. The standoff also had cost Bradley too much, so he sold out to Pittston Coal. The mines continued to produce and still led the county in revenue. Men from Nicholas, Clay, Kanawha and Braxton counties came to make their living in Widen.

It took Joe and Belle half a day to get to Widen on the graveled roads that wound around the ridges. They discussed the events that had been happening at Widen recently and no one seemed to know when or how it would end. When they finally arrived, Belle looked around the streets that were usually overflowing with people. Instead, several houses appeared vacant and neglected. It was quieter now with very few automobiles going through the town and work at a standstill.

Joe's wife Stella was sitting on the porch, fanning herself in the summer heat. Belle could see Stella was glad to see her; she looked like she would give birth very soon. Joe took Belle's bags in the house while Belle stopped to talk with Stella. After they had rested for a while Belle asked Stella when the baby was due. They went into the bedroom and Belle checked her stomach to estimate the weeks until Stella would deliver. She checked her legs and feet for swelling.

Belle believed that the baby would be here soon. Stella and Belle walked down to the neighbor's house and Belle was introduced to the neighbors who were also expecting babies. The first was a young girl named Susie expecting her first baby. She was nervous and that was to be expected. Belle asked some questions and she thought that the baby would probably be due in the next thirty days. Belle said she planned to be here a while, hopefully until the baby arrived.

The other neighbor, June, was sitting on her front porch down the street. June was glad that Belle had come to help them, although June was not due for three months. She was older and she had delivered seven children, so she was not as worried as the other women. Belle told her that she would keep a watch on all three of them while she was here.

Stella was extremely happy to have Belle staying with her. The strike had caused isolation, loneliness, and apprehension to set in. Joe and Stel had wanted to move out, but Joe felt that the strike could end at anytime, and that he should stay and work here. Stel told Belle that people would not believe the violence and crimes that were happening in this coal camp as vigilante justice played out in the cover of darkness. She said that she and Joe kept two loaded guns in their house.

WINTER TIME

It was a cold, hard winter. Belle, George, and Radar had been at home since the snow started in late November. There was a foot of snow on the ground as Belle got dressed to go out and see to her animals. This was the worst winter she had seen in years. Belle put on some long underwear that belonged to George, a pair of pants, tall wool socks, a pullover shirt and a wool sweater. She got her coat buttoned and tied a scarf around her head, putting the scarf tail inside her coat. Finally she put a pair of rubber boots over her shoes and a pair of heavy mittens on her hands. She carried a basket and a bucket and walked carefully on the path that Radar kept shoveled.

The world around Belle was quiet. All one could see was snow everywhere—on the mountains, on the trees, on the ground. It was like living in a bubble; everything and everyone was protecting themselves against the cold. Belle's nose began to freeze before she reached the barn, so she placed her scarf over her face. It was early morning and it must have been below zero. Radar had been doing the chores, but Belle had to get out and breathe some fresh air. They had seen no one and didn't know how others were faring. Belle opened the door to the barn and found her cow standing in its stall. The old cow mooed as Belle patted her. Then Belle pulled some hay and cornstalks for the cow to eat.

When the old cow was quiet, Belle got her three-legged stool and sat down to milk; she got a bucket full and then she found a bowl and poured some warm milk for the barn cats. When she had finished, she placed a clean towel over the bucket and tied it with a string. She went to feed the chickens some cracked corn and gather the eggs. Sixteen eggs—that was a lot for one day. She gathered up her milk and eggs and headed for home. As she walked, she decided she would make some bread pudding today and use some of the eggs. A pan of old bread, some milk, sugar and eggs, a little vanilla cooked into a thick sauce, all mixed together and poured over the bread and baked. Then she would make a sugar glaze and pour it over the hot bread; it would be a nice surprise for supper.

TRAGEDY IN THE WOODS

Summertime had come. Feeling the warmth of the sun and gathering summer fruits renewed people's lives. Word was passed through the neighbors that the Ward Brothers were planning a gathering for the people of the area.

It was set for Saturday night in a large warehouse along the road near Hartland. They planned on singing, square dancing, and feasting. Belle didn't hold with dancing but she liked to visit with neighbors, so she planned to go. Early Saturday she planned her picnic lunch and had it ready to go by noon. They had made plans to ride down with some friends from the other side of the mountain. George and Belle got themselves ready and were waiting on the porch when the old truck sputtered and clanged to a stop by their house. Everyone was in a festive mood as Belle and George crawled in the back of the truck. It was nearly overflowing with children. As the truck slowly traveled down the road they stopped to pick up more people who were walking. It was a jovial day and everyone was in high spirits. When they arrived everyone put the meal together on long tables beneath shade trees along the river. The aroma of food swarmed through the air. They could hear music coming from inside the warehouse and people went in to dance to the banjo, the fiddle and the guitar, kicking up their heels and celebrating life.

The evening wore on and those who did not dance put their chairs under the shade of the trees near the river. They caught up on the news of the community and told who had died, who married and just talked about life in general. As darkness approached, the older women packed up the food and headed for the lantern-lit warehouse. The dancing was the highlight for the young, and the older people sat around the outside walls and watched.

Suddenly the music stopped as a man ran in and began to shout that they needed a doctor. He said a falling tree had hit a man where a crew of loggers was working. The man was outside in a wagon and he had hoped a doctor was near. Belle stepped forward and said, "Young man, I am not a doctor, but I might be able to help until you can get one. Take me to him." Then they hurried outside to see what could be done.

The young man of perhaps thirty years was lying unconscious in the back of a truck; his leg was propped up with coats beneath him. He was going to be in great pain if he came to, so Belle worked quickly. They cut away the pant leg and she ran her hands over the leg to find the broken bones; his thighbone was broken and his knee was shattered. A bone stuck out of the skin below his knee, causing heavy bleeding. Belle wrapped the thighbone with tight strips of cloth and elevated the leg to stop the bleeding. She covered the man with a blanket and told the driver to head for town and a doctor.

Later in the month, a man on crutches got out of a car in front of Belle's house. When she opened the door the man smiled and told her that he came to thank her for helping save his leg. He said, "You probably saved my life and I just had to come and see you." Belle shook his hand and wished him Godspeed. It always felt good when she could help save a life.

BELLE SETS THINGS IN ORDER

"It's a nice day to do some chores around the house," Belle thought, as she walked out to the chicken pen. She was going to feed the chickens and gather the eggs when she heard the hens clucking and fluttering. She dropped her basket and ran to the gate. She knew that some type of thief was visiting. She unlatched the gate and grabbed a piece of steel pipe as she stepped up into the door. A furry varmint swept by her with a hen in its mouth and ran through a hole in the fence. She stepped back and gave a sling of the pipe toward the fox carrying the scared hen. The pipe struck the fox in the head and knocked it out cold; the hen was released from the jaws of death and Belle ran for the gun in her kitchen behind the door. She got close enough to see that the fox was breathing and she gave him one shot to the head. "That will take him to the Pearly Gates," she thought. She turned him over with her foot to make sure he was dead and then she picked him up and gave him a sling into the woods. "That will teach his kind to mess with Belle Neal!" she thought, as he landed in his final resting place. She brushed her hands on her apron and went to repair the hole in the fence. She checked the hen and found only a few teeth marks.

She looked in on the old horse and the milk cow and checked the room over her cellar where two groundhogs lived. She had tamed those crazy groundhogs until they were nearly domestic, spoiled with food and a warm place to spend the winter.

When the weather was right, George and Belle decided they needed to dig a well near their house. They chose the place and contacted a water witch to see if there was any water there before they dug. James Field was known in these mountains as a witcher, good at finding water. He came one day with his peach tree limb and walked around the area they had chosen to dig. He held the bent forked stem out in front of him and walked slowly. When the limb was pulled toward the ground, he marked the spot for water. Belle loved to watch someone do water witchery; it had always fascinated her. They dug the well and had plenty of cold fresh mountain water for years to come.

TWILIGHT YEARS

Belle and George were now in their twilight years; all the children had grown up and moved away to raise families of their own. Radar remained, and he was a great help to Belle. He took over most of the cooking and laundry. As time moved on Radar became pretty much a recluse. Belle still liked to attend church and visit with her families and neighbors, but the years were taking a toll on her. George and Belle were getting too old to walk anywhere, so one summer day, Bib took his sled and his oxen and drove them to his house for a visit and a meal. Marilda's house was always overflowing with family and friends and they were helping to care for their grandchildren while their daughter-in-law Ressa was in the hospital recovering from TB.

When Belle and George were ready to go home, Ruth their niece asked if she could take their picture. They were standing in the road, both bent and old and assisted by canes.

Belle had always been a very outspoken woman, yet she was very aware of children and had great compassion for them. Most did not forget her kind gestures. In 1956 Belle was stricken with a stroke and did not recover. She died at the age of 78; she was born in May and died in May. People around the neighborhood mourned her passing. They were shocked to think that Belle was no longer there. She had been caring for people for so long that it was beyond belief that Belle was gone. She was buried at the Holcomb Cemetery at Bickmore and people came to pay their respects to a woman who devoted so much of her time to the community. Her husband George died soon after Belle, and is buried by her side.

Radar lived alone at the homeplace, living the life of a hermit until eventually some of his family had him placed in an assisted living home in his old age. He remained there until he died. Even to this day if the name Belle Neal is mentioned, someone will recall an event about Belle with a smile on their face.

A NOTE FROM THE AUTHOR

I started working on this book after many years of hearing a great deal about the woman who delivered nearly 3,000 babies in Clay County. Belle Brown Neal was my father's great aunt. We grew up hearing many stories about Aunt Belle and I now live just a short distance from where she lived out her life in a little cabin at the foot of the mountain. Belle died when I was a child of four or or five and while I do not remember seeing her, she had grown larger than life just from all the stories my family told. It seemed that she marched to the beat of a different drum. After working on this book, I can honestly say that she was a radical. She believed in doing things her own way and she did them when she saw fit.

Belle was a legitimate mountain woman, born and raised in these mountains, and she brought up her children during the Great Depression. Through the years that she worked as a granny woman, she helped those who had money for her doctoring as well as those who had nothing. That alone endeared Belle to many. But it was not without reason that she made people furious at her plainspoken ways.

Years ago my high school journalism teacher, Mrs. Jessie Linkinogger, obtained a book for me that I was unable to find; it was about a family in Calhoun County. When I went to her house to pick up the book I told her that I wished someone would write a book about Clay County people and Belle, she said, "You can do it."

I thought, "No, I could never do that!" Mrs. Linkinogger died shortly after my visit and sometimes when I thought of her, I could hear her saying, "You can do it."

This novel is based on the life of Isabel Neal. I spoke with many people who remembered Belle. I put together their accounts of events and elaborated on them. I put her in many situations that very likely did happen during her lifetime. I changed some real names to fiction to avoid offending anyone. Writing this book the past year makes me feel as though I know Belle. Whether people who knew her liked her or not, they would have to say she was unique.

My thanks to my father, Homer Osborne, my Aunt Ann Osborne and my Aunt Ruth Woofter. They told me stories of this woman they held in high regard. I want to thank Belle's granddaughter, Chessie Belle Welch, who allowed me to look at the books Belle used for recording births and for help in portraying Belle as she really was. I also thank my daughter, Shannon Brown, who read the book and made corrections so that the reader could grasp the true meaning of what I put on paper. Sometimes a story would come so fast that I could not put it down quickly enough. She made it legible for you, the reader.

Aunt Belle was part of our family legacy and we were proud to call her our aunt. Belle was genuine as well as unique, and her story needed to be told. Thank you, Aunt .